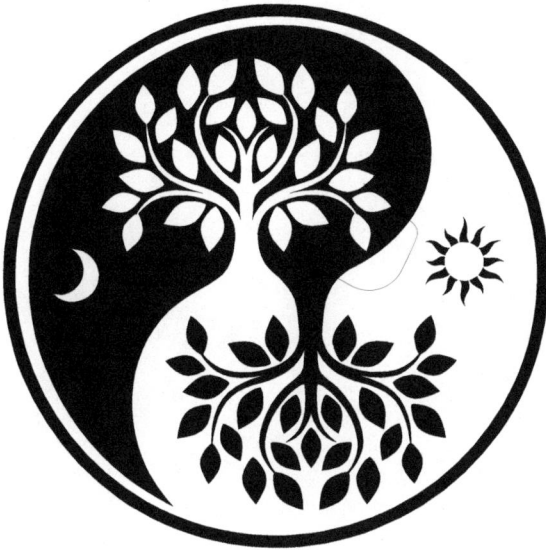

Higher Vibrational Living

Through

Astrology, Essential Oils, and Chinese Medicine

Higher Vibrational Living

First edition July 2018
Printed in the United States of America

Body-Feedback for Health, LLC
2014 Yahara Place, Madison, WI 53704
www.body-feedback.com

For information about special discounts available for bulk purchases, sales promotions, fund-raising, and educational needs, contact Body-Feedback for Health, LLC at 608-535-9144 or info@body-feedback.com.

Visit Michelle Meramour's website www.body-feedback.com
Visit Heather Ensworth's website www.risingmoonhealingcenter.com

Cover design by Jessica Brand
Interior design by Jessica Brand and Body-Feedback For Health, LLC
Illustrations by Body-Feedback For Health, LLC on pages 27, 33, 35, 55, 76, 77, 102, 108, 112, 131, 138, 139, 142, 143, 148, 149, 154, 155, 159, 163, 164, 169, 170, 176, 180, 181, 194, 202, 203, 209, 216, 223, 224, 230, 236, 244, 252, 259, 260, 266, and 273

ISBN 978-0-9992069-0-4 (pbk)
ISBN 978-0-9992069-3-5 (ebook)

Library of Congress Control Number 2017911843
A catalog record for this book is available from the Library of Congress

ACKNOWLEDGMENTS

Michelle and Heather's journey to weave together the common threads of astrology, essential oils, and Chinese medicine required focus, commitment, and patience from a dedicated team believing in the power of personal transformation. We are grateful for those who contributed to all stages of Higher Vibrational Living. First, we are thankful for those who supported us in our vision of integrating these three different approaches to healing. Next, we are grateful for the team of professionals who helped bring form and beauty to the sentences we carefully crafted. And finally, we are thankful for the team that assisted with the publishing process. We acknowledge the cooperative efforts of the many people who came together to bring life to this work.

Most importantly, we would like to thank our clients and students whose journeys to develop better health emotionally and spiritually and to raise their consciousness inspired us to create this work and share it with the world.

With love,
Michelle and Heather

TABLE OF CONTENTS

Allie's Transformation

Allie, a thirty-seven-year-old, career-driven woman on her second marriage, felt incomplete and dissatisfied even though certain areas of her life were going well. She had graduated from college and after a few entry-level jobs went to work for a large company with high demands, constant stress, and very little job satisfaction. After ten years of this lifestyle, she became depressed, lacked enthusiasm, and was physically burned out. Due to the constant stress, Allie began to experience hormonal imbalances, such as irregular cycles, moodiness, acne, skin irritations, and other symptoms of PMS—all of which left her feeling self-conscious and reduced her ability to enjoy everyday life.

Both of Allie's parents had been self-employed entrepreneurs for most of their lives. Her mother gave up her small retail shop, which she thoroughly enjoyed, to work for a large hospital when Allie was a teenager. The hospital provided job security, health insurance, and retirement benefits that she lacked being self-employed. But Allie noticed a change in her mother over time; she grew pessimistic and lost her zest for life. It became increasingly clear that the job left her mother unfulfilled. Allie realized that she was reliving her mother's unhappiness and that the career path she had chosen was stifling her ability to express her true self. It was leading her further away from her heart's desire: to be an entrepreneur in the healing arts. Allie imagined her mother must have felt a similar loss many years ago.

Allie decided to try acupuncture with Michelle to address her physical and emotional symptoms. During their work together, Michelle recommended using essential oils timed with Allie's menstrual cycle to support specific hormones at the proper time. Allie's hormones balanced quickly. Her cycles became regular, her acne and skin cleared up, and her mood stabilized. Allie felt better about herself and found joy in other activities outside of her career.

Allie saw Michelle every few months for acupuncture sessions to keep up her improved health. One day, Michelle mentioned a new approach she'd developed which combined specific essential oil blends with a person's astrological birth information. This piqued Allie's curiosity, and she agreed to let Michelle make recommendations based on her astrology chart. After working with these new blends for a few months, Allie saw what needed to change in her life to set her on a career path that spoke to her soul.

Prior to working with Michelle, Allie had no experience using an astrology chart or understanding how to work with essential oils based on it. She used the free astrology chart services offered online to learn about her sun and moon signs and her Ascendant along with her planetary influences. Allie studied the basics of her astrological natal (birth) chart and over time these skills became second nature. She related with the astrological information she read about herself and trusted her intuition to choose the essential oil blends to work with each day.

Allie consulted with Heather to do a more in-depth astrology reading to understand herself and her chart more fully. The astrology reading that Allie experienced with Heather confirmed that Allie's intuition about changing her career path was right for her. Allie had felt a strong attraction to do work in the healing arts for years. The reading helped her to make sense of why she felt this way, and it provided reassurance that the steps she was taking were on her true path.

Over the next year, Allie experienced insight and confirmation of her intuitions and decisions as she explored her astrological influences. Allie's self-discovery process included creating a plan of action to change careers. She believed the astrology blends gave her support to make the needed changes. She said, "It felt like a calling from my higher self or the Divine to live a more meaningful and self-expressed life." Taking the time to understand her chart, using the astrology blends on a daily basis, and continuing her monthly acupuncture sessions helped Allie harness the planetary influences that created the catalyst for change. She continues to feel improved emotional and physical health. For the first time in her life, Allie says she feels aligned with her true self.

According to Allie, the changes she experienced have been profound. She gained confidence, self-worth, and inner peace. From this vantage point, she discovered what really made her happy, what her gifts were, and what she wanted to do with her career. Allie now has a level of certainty that she is on the right path and can make major career changes. She trusts that everything is going to work out, and she is no longer making important decisions based on avoiding risks and worrying that she is not good enough to be a successful entrepreneur.

By combining the elements of acupuncture, essential oil blends, and astrological information, Allie experienced higher vibrational living. For her, higher vibrational living manifested in trusting and following her inner guidance and gaining the confidence needed to take on new opportunities to expand her body, mind, and spirit. Allie's deeper understanding of her astrology chart, combined with her use of the astrological essential oil blends, encouraged a better understanding of her true nature. The oils worked on an energetic level while she consciously processed the information she was learning about herself. She gained trust in herself and her connection with Spirit. She felt energetically lighter and experienced healthier interactions with her husband, community, and everyone with whom she came in contact.

With a new sense of confidence, Allie negotiated reduced hours at her corporate job. Finally, she had the freedom and the time needed for self-discovery and to follow her heart's desires as a yoga instructor and entrepreneur. After thirteen years in Corporate America, ten of them knowing she would never be happy working in this environment, she was able to take the leap of faith and enjoy the process of transformation and self-discovery. Six months after she reduced her hours at her job, Allie ended her corporate career and expanded her entrepreneurial ventures and her work as a yoga instructor to full-time.

There is no passion to be found playing small – in settling for a life that is less than the one you are capable of living.

—Nelson Mandela

Higher Vibrational Living for You

Higher vibrational living means something different to everyone, and your path is as unique as your fingerprint. Self-discovery, self-love, and understanding pave the way for growth, self-expression, and healthy relationships. Wherever you are along your journey, this book will provide a new understanding, perspectives, and tools to improve your daily life. By gaining insight and bringing a new level of awareness to your decisions, you can grow and transform areas of your life where you feel blocked or stuck as well as enhancing your gifts and strengths.

In this book, you will learn how to:

- Look up your birth chart and determine your sun and moon signs along with challenging and beneficial planetary aspects

- Understand how your sun and moon signs with their planetary aspects reflect your identity, strengths and weaknesses, and emotional nature, and learn how they influence your physical and emotional health

- Choose essential oil blends designed to help you come into balance and gain insight about yourself by harmonizing with the challenging and beneficial aspects in your astrological chart

- Utilize different methods of applying essential oils to balance your acupuncture meridian system and thereby support both physical and emotional health

- Use affirmations with your essential oils to enhance their benefits as well as to gain increased awareness and to focus on your inherent strengths

- Access the wisdom of modern astrology and ancient Chinese medicine to harmonize and empower who you are physically, emotionally, and spiritually

This book will guide you step by step through the process of understanding your astrology chart, using essential oils based on your chart, and applying them to balance your acupuncture meridian system. If you are new astrology, essential oils, or Chinese medicine, this book will provide a solid foundation to access these healing modalities. If you are knowledgeable in one or more of these areas, this process will open up a new dimension of self-awareness and transformation.

A New Paradigm of Energy Medicine

If you want to find the secrets of the universe,
think in terms of energy, frequency, and vibration.

—Nikola Tesla

A new model of energy medicine is offered here to guide you on a path of self-discovery and to empower you to engage in your own healing process, live in a more balanced way, and move more fully into your gifts and the uniqueness of who you are. This new model blends the wisdom of Western astrology, the practices of Chinese medicine, and the healing potential of essential oils to help you to restore balance and harmony. Together, astrology and traditional Chinese medicine guide you in understanding how to come into balance and wholeness.

Both modern Western astrology and ancient Chinese philosophy explore the energies of nature and the seasonal cycle and how these relate to energy patterns in our bodies. Both systems are based on the understanding that health and wholeness are related to our being in balance in our bodies and in harmony with the energies of the natural world. Working with the aspects in your astrology chart, the seasonal energies, and the acupuncture meridians (energy circuits), you can assess your challenges, strengths, and vulnerabilities, and gain understanding in how to move into balance and wholeness. You can then apply the astrology oil blends to promote harmony in your life and raise your energy vibration. Woven together, these modalities will support you in healing and coming into the fullness of who you are—physically, emotionally, and spiritually.

As was known in ancient wisdom traditions, and now has been proven by quantum physics, our bodies consist of energy and are affected by the energies that surround us. To be healthy, it is important to be in balance and harmony within yourself, in your relationships with others, and in your relationship with the natural environment.

Often physical symptoms or illnesses are messages to you that your life is out of balance in some way. Emotional problems may be alerting you to issues that need healing or to ways in which you are out of alignment with your true self.

When you consciously integrate these messages and work to clear blocks and rebalance yourself at the energetic level, the process supports healing at the physical and emotional levels. In this way, healing occurs as an integrative process including the physical, emotional, and spiritual aspects of who you are. To be healthy and whole means to be true to who you uniquely are, to be in alignment with your true nature, and to be in balance and in harmony within yourself, your relationships, and the natural environment.

Western astrology arises from the ancient wisdom that the energies of the Earth mirror the energies of the sky. Everything is a part of the interconnected web of life. Who you are is shaped by the energies present at the moment of your birth. What you do with those energy patterns is your choice. You have free will. Astrology is not deterministic. An understanding of the astrological patterns helps guide you in understanding yourself more fully and living at a higher evel of consciousness and energy vibration. Through understanding the energy patterns in your birth chart, and especially the energies of your Sun (essence) and Moon (emotional nature), you can step into the fullness of who you are and live in a conscious way, in balance within yourself and with the cosmos.

To be in balance from an astrological perspective is to live your life consciously and to be aware of the different facets of who you are through understanding the energies of your Sun and Moon and their aspects with planetary energies. It involves integrating these energies so that you are working with the gifts of the themes in your chart rather than having facets of yourself in conflict with each other or living in an unconscious or reactive way. To be out of balance is to be unaware of parts of yourself, to be in conflict with aspects of who you are, or to be living your life in a reactive or unconscious manner.

Traditional Chinese medicine provides a proven template of your body's energy system, which influences your physical, emotional, and spiritual health. This ancient healing tradition is also attuned to the seasonal cycle and how the energies of the natural environment affect your health. Traditional Chinese medicine works at the energetic level to restore balance to the body and to help you live in harmony with the rhythms and cycles of the seasons and with your own energy patterns.

Essential oils raise your energetic frequency and vibrational level to facilitate emotional, physical, and spiritual healing. Essential oils are the lifeblood of plants; they transport nutrients, oxygen, and enzymes for the plant to grow and heal. Essential oils vibrate at a very high energy level, helping your body to release toxins and imbalances, to heal, and to return to inner harmony.

In this book, you will learn how to use your birth chart to see what life themes you are dealing with, what challenges and vulnerabilities you have, and how to honor your true self. You will be guided in how to integrate the aspects in your astrology chart with the associated Chinese medicine meridians and organ systems and how to apply the proper essential oils to support you in your healing and transformation. Using this integration of astrology, Chinese medicine, and essential oils, you can support yourself in coming into harmony and balance physically, emotionally, and spiritually. You will also learn how to raise your vibrational level to break free from old, unhealthy patterns and move into a higher level of consciousness. You will find a path to healing and personal transformation through increasing your self-awareness, raising your vibrational level, and coming into balance and wholeness.

If you are interested in further information about the history of astrology, Chinese medicine, and the use of essential oils for healing, please see the appendix starting on page 279.

How the Authors Came to Develop this New Paradigm

Heather Ensworth, an astrologer and clinical psychologist, has studied many ancient wisdom and healing traditions, and how these traditions give us greater insight into ways to address our current emotional and physical imbalances. She integrates astrology and psychology and uses her clients' birth charts and current planetary influences to provide them with a deeper understanding of themselves and to support them in their unique healing process. Challenging aspects in people's birth charts and the current transits often relate to the emotional and physical issues that people experience. By gaining insight about these energy patterns, it is possible for people to have a better understanding of the difficulties they face and how to move into balance and harmony so healing may occur.

Prior to becoming an acupuncturist, Michelle Meramour studied Western astrology and came to realize how planetary influences affect health. She now practices one of the oldest styles of acupuncture known today. The earliest written acupuncture texts looked to current planetary influences to predict health challenges in general. Over her years of practice, Michelle studied the correlations between the challenging aspects in the birth chart, transits, seasonal shifts, and the associated meridian or organ imbalances.

In collaborating, both Michelle and Heather realized that at the heart of both Chinese medicine and Western astrology is a recognition of how the energies of the Earth and sky affect our lives and guide us in ways we can heal. Their shared passion for an integrative healing approach naturally encouraged working together with mutual clients and then expanded into teaching classes together.

Together, Michelle and Heather researched the ancient Chinese medical texts to find the original connections between the Chinese astrological system and meridian theory. They then explored how these connections weave together the ancient Chinese understanding with the modern Western astrological system through their similar understanding of the interactions between the energies of the sky and Earth, of the seasonal cycles, and of our bodies.

This overlay of the corresponding meridians on the astrological wheel yielded outstanding results with clients. Clients reported that this integrated approach released physical tension and pain and supported both physical and emotional healing.

During this period of collaboration, Michelle also created two types of essential oil blends: the meridian-balancing/planetary blends and the organ-supporting/astrology sign blends. The first set of blends effectively addresses both meridian imbalances and planetary influences. By weaving together the aspects in the birth chart and the Chinese meridian and organ systems, a valuable paradigm developed for understanding the roots of emotional and physical issues that compromise health. Clients who incorporated this new treatment approach with the other modalities they were using experienced deep healing on all levels: physically, emotionally, and spiritually.

The use of essential oils for physical and emotional healing along with spiritual transformation is just as ancient as astrology and traditional Chinese medicine. Essential oils carry the highest vibration in the natural medicine world and contain oxygen, which makes them the lifeblood of plants and powerful tools for physical, emotional, and spiritual healing. They even produce biophotons, which emit low levels of ultraviolet light that in turn influence many cellular functions. Many pioneers in holistic medicine believe essential oils hold the potential to support the expanding spiritual consciousness on our planet.

The life force in everything can be measured by electrical frequencies that give off a specific vibration. For example, organic fresh vegetables and sprouted grains have the highest electrical frequencies or vibration among foods, while canned and processed foods hold little to no electrical frequency and carry a very low vibration. When your electrical vibration is high, you feel energized, positive, and generally upbeat. When your electrical vibration is low, you feel lethargic and emotionally off-balance. Emotional upsets, negative internal dialogue, and illness will lower the vibrational frequencies of your body. Therapeutic-grade essential oils carry high electrical frequencies and raise the vibration of whatever they come into contact with.

As Michelle and Heather collaborated and worked with this integration of astrology, Chinese medicine, and essential oils, a new highly effective paradigm of energy medicine emerged that supports healing on all levels and increases self-awareness, balance, and energetic vibration. As you work with this paradigm, you can explore how this integrative approach will help you heal and come into balance, and how it will support you in moving into the fullness of who you are.

Western Astrology and Chinese Medicine

Western Astrology and the Chinese Energy Almanac

The Ten Heavenly Stems and Twelve Earthly Branches

The primary connection between the Western astrological wheel and traditional Chinese medicine is their association with the seasonal cycle. The similarities of the seasonal cycle described by both Western astrologers tracking the signs of the zodiac around the wheel and the ancient Chinese acupuncturists describing the twelve earthly branches (seasonal months) are amazingly alike. Both track the energy changes on Earth as the Sun moves through the sky in its annual cycle. Both understand that the patterns in the heavens mirror the energies and events on the Earth ("as above, so below"). Both relate the influences of the seasonal cycle to specific effects on people's physical and emotional health.

As the Sun circles around the wheel, it energizes different signs and sections of the chart in its annual cycle. Likewise, as the Sun moves through the twelve earthly branches (seasonal months), it affects different aspects of health, related to specific times of the year and the associated meridians and organs.

The Wheel of the Year in Western Astrology

The Western astrological wheel of the year begins with Aries on the Ascendant and proceeds in a counterclockwise direction (see the diagram below). The signs reflect the seasonal cycle and correlate with the four elements in traditional astrology (earth, air, fire, and water) and the three modalities (cardinal, mutable, and fixed), which relate to the flow of energies through the seasons. The cardinal signs mark the beginning of a new season, while the fixed signs signify the consolidation and full expression of that season, and the mutable signs show the transition into the next season. The cardinal signs also mark the solstices and equinoxes, while the fixed signs hold the anciently sacred "cross-quarter" holidays that are the midpoints between the solstices and equinoxes.

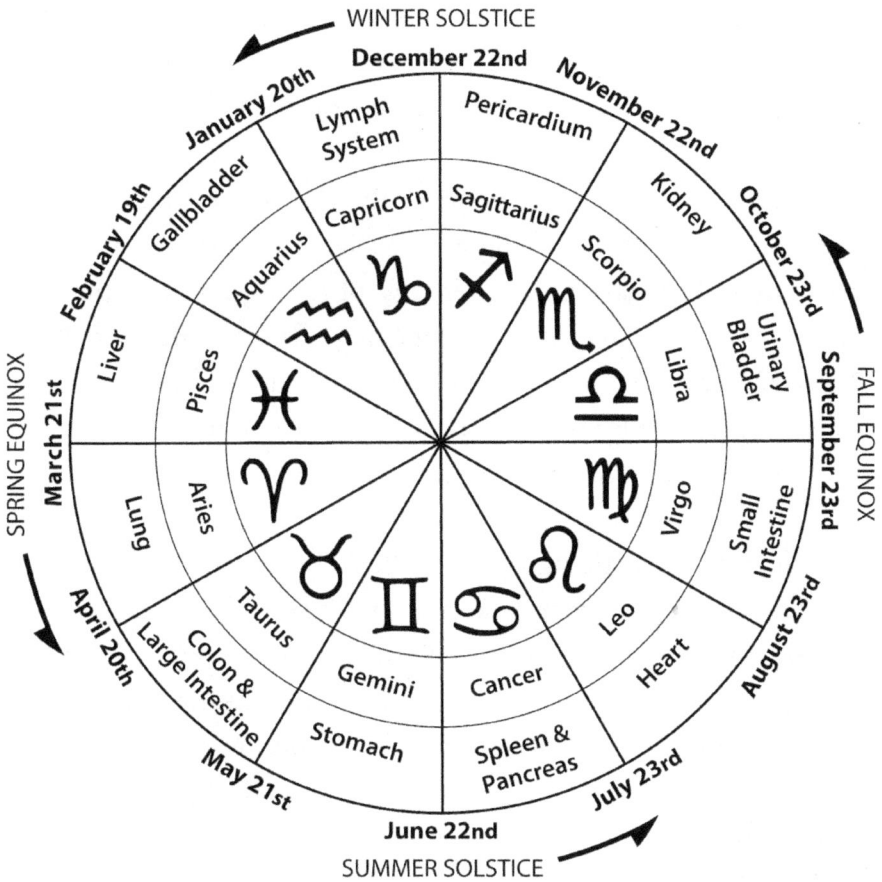

The Astrological Wheel of the Year for the Northern Hemisphere

Below are descriptions of the seasons and signs of the Western astrological wheel.

SPRING:

Aries, a cardinal fire sign, initiates the season of spring with the heat and outward energy of new beginnings after the inward quality of winter. Aries begins with the spring equinox when the day and night are equal in length; and then, following the equinox, the light increases with the movement into spring. The sign of Aries and the direction of EAST are associated with the Ascendant of the chart. Planetary ruler: Mars

Taurus, a fixed earth sign, displays the full manifestation of the colors and textures of spring as the plants and trees come into full bloom. This is when the energy of spring consolidates and manifests in its fullness. The ancient holiday of Beltane (May Day) occurs during Taurus and is the midpoint between the spring equinox and summer solstice. This was the time when the beauty and fertility of the Earth were celebrated. Planetary ruler: Venus

Gemini, a mutable air sign, marks the transition from spring into summer and is the season when the pollinators (bees, butterflies, and hummingbirds) come to distribute the energy of the plants and foster growth. Gemini carries the energy of making connections and spreading the seeds of life. Planetary ruler: Mercury

SUMMER:

Cancer, a cardinal water sign, begins the season of summer with the summer solstice, the longest day of the year. The sign of Cancer is in the NORTH and is when the Sun moves to its most northern position in relation to the equator of the Earth. In the natural wheel of the year, this sign is associated with the root of the chart (known as the IC or Imum Coeli). Ruler: Moon

Leo, a fixed fire sign, holds the fullness of the energy of summer and the heat of the Sun. This fixed sign consolidates the energy of summer and marks the ancient Lammas festival (August 1st) honoring the midpoint between the summer solstice and fall equinox. Ruler: Sun

Virgo, a mutable earth sign, signifies the transition from summer into fall with the harvest and reaping of what was grown through spring and summer. This is the time of year for "separating the wheat from the chaff" and storing the fruits of the harvest in preparation for the winter. Planetary ruler: Mercury

AUTUMN:

Libra, a cardinal air sign, begins the autumn season with the fall equinox when the energies of day and night again come into balance. The sign of Libra is in the WEST and is on the Descendant in the natural wheel of the year. Planetary ruler: Venus

Scorpio, a fixed water sign, signifies the increasing hours of darkness and the deepening of the energy of autumn when the trees lose their leaves and the energy of the Earth pulls in its life force. Scorpio marks the midpoint (November 1st) between the fall equinox and the winter solstice with the ancient sacred festival of Samhain. This was a ceremonial event to honor ancestors and those who have died and to honor the end of the harvest and the dying back of the plants before winter. The remnants of this ancient holiday are present in the celebration of Halloween and All Saints Day. Modern planetary ruler: Pluto

Sagittarius, a mutable fire sign, marks the transition into winter and was the time, in ancient cultures, when people would gather around the fire in the growing cold and darkness to tell stories and prepare for the coming of winter. As the darkness increases, it is also a time for being more aware of the stars and seeking guidance from above. Planetary ruler: Jupiter

WINTER:

Capricorn, a cardinal earth sign, initiates the movement into the season of winter with the winter solstice, the longest night and shortest day of the year. This is the time when the energy of the Earth moves inward, and the seeds and plants are in hibernation awaiting the coming of spring. It marks the direction of SOUTH and is when the Sun is in its southernmost placement in the sky. In the natural wheel of the year, Capricorn is on the Midheaven. Planetary ruler: Saturn

Aquarius, a fixed air sign, occurs during the heart of winter and the season of snow and ice in the northern hemisphere. Aquarius signifies the energy of the increasing light at this time of year. This fixed sign holds the midpoint between the winter solstice and spring equinox (February 1st) with the ancient festival of Imbolc. This was a time for divination and seeking guidance for the coming year. Modern planetary ruler: Uranus

Pisces, a mutable water sign, is the last sign in the wheel of the year. Pisces reflects the ending of winter and the transition into spring with the coming of the rains and the melting of snow, increasing the flow of the rivers and streams. Modern planetary ruler: Neptune

The Ten Heavenly Stems and Twelve Earthly Branches

Many ancient cultures and current indigenous cultures believe that everything is created from and in relationship with the World Tree, which bridges the energy of the Earth and sky. Modern science is now seeing evidence of this energetic tree of life in the cosmos. The ancient Chinese described this bridge of energy as "ten heavenly stems" and "twelve earthly branches."

The ten heavenly stems relate to the five elements (wood, fire, earth, metal, and water), the five seasons of the year (spring, summer, late summer, fall, winter), and the five directions (east, south, west, north, and center). The stems also reflect the primary constellations in the sky, which are considered to mirror the elements and five directions.

The twelve earthly branches relate to the twelve months of the year and the corresponding growth cycles of vegetation. The twelve meridians and their two-hour segments of a twenty-four hour day relate to the twelve earthly branches. Together, the heavenly stems and earthly branches integrate the energy flow, or weather patterns, between the Earth and the sky. The integration of the heavenly stems and earthly branches creates five sixty-year cycles, representing the twelve animals of the Chinese zodiac with each of the five elements. These sixty-year cycles are the basis for the Chinese calendar.

Acupuncturists commonly see organ weaknesses exacerbated based on the change of season and, more specifically during the change of the astrological sign within that season. Supporting different organs based on the seasons is a common practice among acupuncturists.

For more information on the integration of Chinese medicine with Western astrology and the seasonal cycle, please see page 292 of the appendix.

The Chinese Medicine Clock

According to Chinese Medicine, energy peaks in each of the twelve organs and its associated meridian every two hours, to complete a full circuit in twenty-four hours or one day, as depicted in the following diagram. The daily circulation of the acupuncture meridian system begins at 3 a.m. with the lung meridian. Each organ is most active during its two-hour period, and each meridian circulates into the next in a clockwise pattern. For example, the colon and large intestine meridian are most active between 5 a.m. and 7 a.m., releasing stool from yesterday's digestive process. The stomach organ and meridian are most active from 7 a.m. to 9 a.m. to process the first stage of digestion for the most important meal of the day, breakfast.

Throughout each day, the energy moves through the Chinese clock, activating the corresponding meridians and organs in the diurnal cycle. How your body responds to the increase in energy depends on how balanced the meridian is and how the season and planetary aspects influence that particular meridian. Planetary aspects can be either beneficial or challenging to a specific meridian, based on your natal birth chart and the current position of the planets in the sky. Depending on several factors, you may find this energy either easy or challenging to process physically or emotionally.

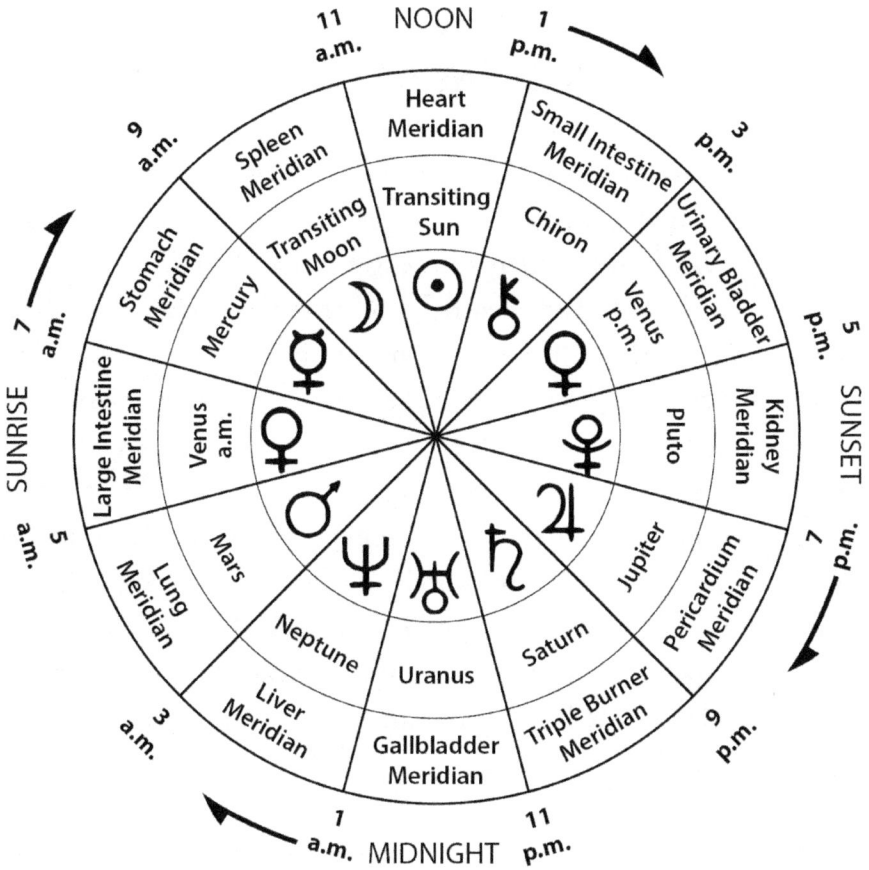

The Chinese Medicine Clock

The Astrological Wheel and the Chinese Medicine Clock

Though the Astrological Wheel and the Chinese Medicine Clock circle in different directions, they both follow the same progression through the body's corresponding organs and meridians. Moreover, Michelle and Heather find that the astrological signs correlate with the Chinese organ systems, and the planetary rulers of each sign correlate with the Chinese medicine meridians. Inverting the direction of either the wheel or the clock will bring the two diagrams into sync with each other, making it easier to see the correlations. For example, segment A of the Astrological Wheel is the sign of Aries, which is ruled by the planet Mars, and corresponds to Mars in segment A of the Chinese Medicine Clock. Likewise, segment B of the Astrological wheel is the sign of Taurus, which is ruled by Venus a.m. in segment B of the Chinese Medicine Clock. And so forth.

Despite these close correlations, however, the two systems differ somewhat in their understanding of health issues. From the Western astrology perspective, the signs of the zodiac correlate primarily with the physical aspects of the body, from Aries at the head to Pisces at the feet. Western astrology is more symptom-focused while Chinese medicine is more focused on the interconnectedness of the body and its energy systems.

The emotions that relate to the organs in Chinese medicine are associated with the archetypal energies of the signs because of their similarities. For example, if someone's lung organ energy is compromised, they find it challenging to receive direction from their source or higher-self at a steady pace. The emotions relating to the meridians are associated with the planets because

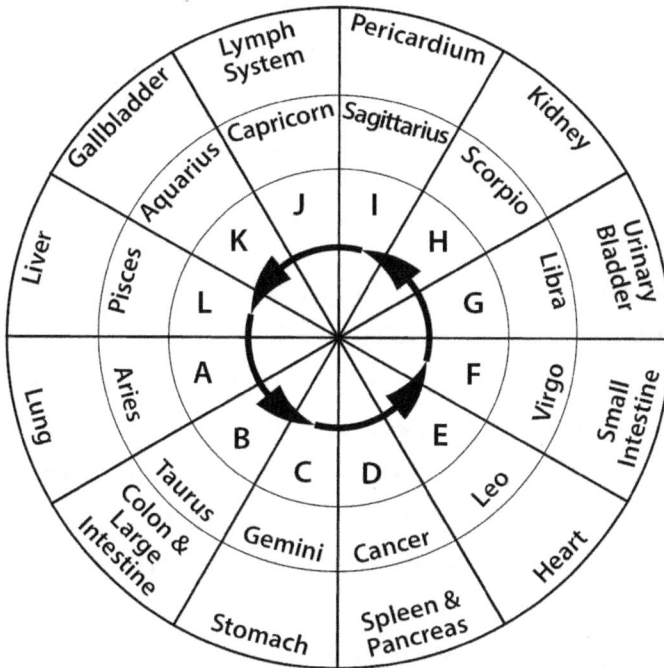

The Astrological Wheel circles counter-clockwise

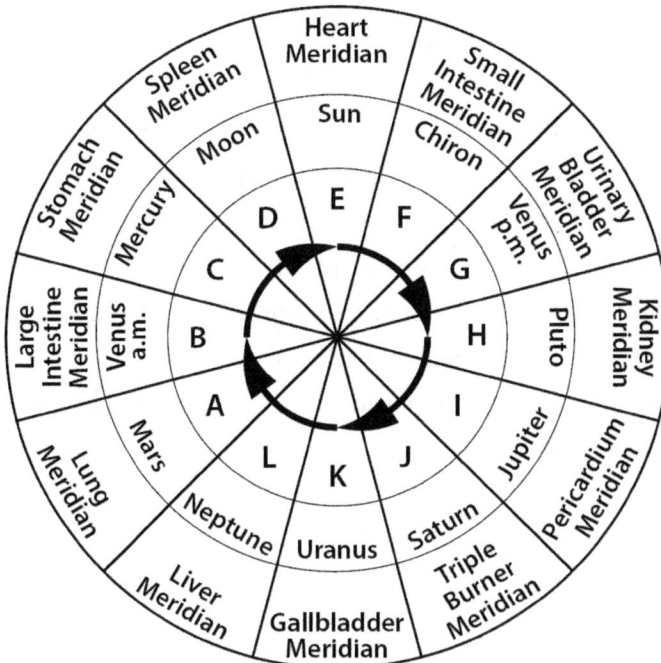

The Chinese Medicine Clock circles clockwise

of their similarities. For example, if someone's lung meridian is imbalanced, they struggle with healthy boundaries, and they become hot-tempered easily. In summary, a sign correlates with the Chinese organ while it's planetary ruler corresponds with that organ's meridian.

In general, the bio-energetic and emotional aspects of the meridians and organs correlate more closely with the archetypal meanings and energies of the planets and signs rather than the physical attributes. The chart on page 286 of the appendix summarizes the major correlations between Chinese medicine meridians and the Western astrology ruling planets, along with their associated medical functions or physiological and bio-energetic processes.

It is valuable to see how the two systems correlate as well as to honor their differences. As you work with the connections between the planets and meridians and signs of the zodiac and Chinese organ systems, allow yourself to integrate their similarities and also their differences. Both Chinese medicine and astrology are based on a belief that the heavenly influences and seasonal changes affect your physical and emotional health. While Western astrologers and modern acupuncturists approach this synthesis in different ways, both systems hold the awareness that everything is interconnected. As you begin to work with your personal chart, you will support your health and well-being by aligning with the energy patterns of the Earth and sky to feel physically, emotionally, and spiritually balanced.

Energy Medicine and the Blending of Astrology, Acupuncture, and Essential Oils

Energy medicine supports healing by bringing us back into balance and harmony within ourselves and in our relationship with the Earth and sky and the cycles of the seasons. Traditional Chinese medicine places emphasis on harmonizing constitutional organ imbalances to support optimal health. Acupuncturists often refer to this as the "root pattern of imbalance"; by correcting this, the body can self-heal, and symptoms naturally improve.

Constitutional organ imbalances often correspond with difficult astrological Sun and Moon natal aspects and in genetic tendencies seen in the father's or mother's health. In Western astrology, the natal Sun and Moon correspond with our sense of self, health, and emotional nature. Also, the Sun and Moon in the chart indicate how we experienced our parents' influence both emotionally and physically.

In traditional Chinese medicine, a common practice is to support the organs based on the seasonal cycle. For example, spring allergies triggered by the melting snow and budding trees in late March and early April will negatively affect lung function and may cause shortness of breath, chronic cough, itchy throat and eyes, postnasal drip, and sneezing. Excessive fluid retention, with swollen ankles and fingers, loose stools, and low energy, affects the spleen organ and is naturally worse in late June and early July when the humidity is highest from spring showers and damp environments. Acupuncturists find that supporting the associated organ during the corresponding season helps the body to adjust to the weather changes and promotes a strong constitution.

When the Sun passes through a particular sign of the zodiac during the season, you might feel energized and rejuvenated if you have harmonious aspects to that part of your chart, or you will feel depleted and weak with difficult or challenging aspects. The exact time of birth, birthplace, and aspects in the natal chart determine the personal interaction with the season. This will be discussed in more depth later, but harmonious aspects tend to be conjunctions, sextiles, or trines, while challenging aspects are usually squares or oppositions.

Because of the relationship of the acupuncture meridian system to the seasonal cycle and the diurnal cycle, constitutional imbalances can also trigger symptoms at specific times of the day, which correspond with the two-hour period influenced by the meridian. The most challenged meridian and corresponding time of day relate with the most challenging planetary aspects to the natal Sun or Moon in the birth chart. When the time of day energizes a particular meridian and sign, it also stimulates the corresponding planetary ruler in the birth chart. Many people find their symptoms flare up if the time of day is energizing a challenging aspect to the natal Sun or Moon. They tend to feel best when the time of day stimulates a harmonious aspect.

Acupuncturists look for symptoms that occur at a specific time of day, as well as specific times in the seasonal cycle, and work to harmonize the two meridians or organs that are opposite each other to relieve those particular symptoms. In Chinese medicine, every physical imbalance has a corresponding emotional challenge. Understanding your basic natal chart provides insights into both physical and emotional health and shows how you can navigate challenges and embrace your strengths in life.

From a Western astrology perspective, challenging aspects to the Sun, Moon, or Ascendant show ongoing issues that you may be dealing with, either physically or emotionally. Challenging aspects to the Sun often indicate difficulties affecting your sense of self, constitution, or energy level. In relationship with the Moon, these challenging aspects are likely to manifest in either health issues or emotional difficulties. On the Ascendant, challenging aspects may indicate birth trauma, chronic physical or emotional issues, or problematic dynamics in relationships with others. Other challenging aspects or difficult configurations in certain houses in the astrological chart may highlight particular areas of stress in your life. When the current transits activate one of these challenging aspects or houses, these issues are likely to flare up or become more acute.

It is also possible to see indications of genetic issues in the chart (in challenging aspects on the root of the chart or to the Sun or Moon) as well as karmic issues. Challenges to the Sun and Moon and possible associated emotional and physical challenges are discussed in detail throughout this book. Difficulties related to past life trauma are seen in the placements of Pluto, Uranus, and the lunar nodes in the chart, but are too advanced to cover in this book. (For further information about this, read Jeffrey Wolf Green's book, *Pluto: The Evolutionary Journey of the Soul*, Volume 1.)

As we work with these challenging aspects or transits in a conscious way, they become areas of growth and evolution. From her years of clinical experience and astrological readings, Heather has seen that working with these challenges in the chart in an unconscious manner causes them to likely manifest at a physical level. When we work with them with awareness, then these challenging aspects or transits are more likely to manifest at an emotional level. When we live at a higher spiritual level, these challenging aspects or transits tend to lead to transformation and emotional and spiritual evolution. However, genetic, family lineage patterns, or karmic issues may manifest in a physical way even for those of us who are highly conscious; this may indicate deeper karmic or family patterns that need to be healed and cleared at all levels. We also live in a world that is out of balance with the seasonal cycle and with the natural world, which exposes us to toxins and stresses our immune systems and health. As we come more into balance, we experience a more harmonious relationship with the world around us, which supports our healing and the healing of the environment.

Understanding the harmonious aspects in the chart helps you become aware of your natural gifts and strengths. Working with the challenging aspects in a conscious way supports you in growing and developing emotionally and spiritually. As the planets move through the solar system, they create configurations in interaction with your chart (known as "transits") that can be either supportive or challenging and are catalysts or messengers, bringing unresolved issues to consciousness for healing and transformation.

Essential oils are the perfect self-care tool because they are versatile and support both physical and emotional health and spiritual evolution. The sign and planetary oil blends harmonize your astrological influences and planetary aspects with the seasonal and the diurnal cycles. These same blends support healthy organ and acupuncture meridian functions. Harmonizing your meridian system and the aspects in your birth chart helps you to stay in balance and live at your highest potential.

Application Methods
for Essential Oils

Essential oils provide an immediate energetic shift by crossing the blood-brain barrier and affecting the whole body. Upon inhalation, essential oils activate neurons found in the sinuses that send information directly to several areas of the brain. The sense of smell is the only one of our five senses that has direct pathways to the frontal lobe, temporal lobe, limbic system, and hippocampus. These areas have a powerful influence on our health, personalities, emotions, and on our perceptions of happiness.

Because therapeutic grade essential oils quickly penetrate the brain, they can potentially affect almost every system in the body. Essential oils are the only natural substances that cross the blood-brain barrier to bring nutrients and oxygen to the brain, the body's command center.

Using essential oils with intention and gratitude supports your commitment to higher vibrational living. Showing gratitude for the essential oils honors their gifts and healing properties. Gratitude itself shifts your energy to a higher vibration and increases the healing benefits of the essential oils. The carefully crafted affirmations included in this book can support you in using your oils consciously and help to improve their healing benefits.

Diffusing Essential Oils

Diffusing therapeutic-grade essential oils creates a constant release of tiny, high-vibrating molecules that enter the brain to balance emotions and relieve stress instantly. Whatever the nature of the stress, diffusing essential oils is beneficial. It is especially helpful to diffuse the astrological sign blends during their corresponding time of the year to help you harmonize with the current seasonal cycle. When you first begin diffusing essential oils, it is best to start slowly. Diffuse oils for ten to twenty minutes every two to three hours. Children are easily adaptable and respond well to twenty minutes of oils diffused a couple of times a day. Non-diluted essential oils are best for diffusing as the essential oil molecule disperses into the water vapor and releases into the air. Adding vegetable oils to therapeutic-grade essential oils creates particles too dense to effectively vaporize and the oil residue coats the diffuser.

Therapeutic grade essential oil diffusers use either cold air or cold water to break down the tiny molecules in the oils, dispersing them slowly into the air. This atomization keeps the oil in the air for hours after being diffused. Water-based diffusers can run with fewer drops of oils for longer periods of time than cold-air diffusers because the essential oils are first dispersed in the water to dilute them. Water-based diffusers usually have an automatic shut-off when the water runs out. You can adjust the number of drops mixed with the water based on the size of the room and desired intensity. Diffusing essential oils directly, without diluting them in water, causes the oil to spread faster and works best in damp or humid climates or where there are issues with mold.

You can make your own manual diffuser using a glass spray bottle and four to six drops of essential oil per ounce of distilled water. This application method works best when using undiluted essential oils as a perfume or room spray and will help your oils last longer. Smaller spray bottles are ideal for travel, and a few sprays can raise the frequency everywhere you go. A small amount of an essential oil can go a long way when mixed with water in a glass spray bottle.

Heating essential oils using candles or burners is not recommended. This eliminates the healing properties of the therapeutic-grade essential oils and can actually release toxic chemicals into your immediate environment.

Topical Application of Essential Oils

How often you need to apply the oils and how many drops you use is a personal preference. You can quickly set a positive intention for the day by applying your essential oils with the sign or planetary affirmations provided in later sections of this book.

Vegetable oils (such as olive, almond, jojoba, or avocado) safely dilute essential oils. Water actually drives the essential oils deeper into the tissue, making them feel more intense. As you experiment with different application sites, if a particular oil or oil blend feels too hot, rub some vegetable oil on top of it instead of trying to wash it off.

Skin reactions may occur if you have used or are now using beauty products containing toxic chemicals. Skin irritation can happen when essential oils break down the toxic residue left in the skin layer. Chemicals that tend to create the most reactions when mixed with essential oils include synthetic fragrances (phthalates), synthetic colors, parabens, ureas, propylene and polyethylene glycols, sodium lauryl sulfate, MEA (monoethanolamine), DEA (diethanolamine), and TEA (triethanolamine). If you have used or are now using any of these chemicals and are experiencing skin reactions, we recommend working with a licensed holistic health-care provider to create a balanced long-term cleanse that detoxifies the skin.

Certain essential oils can increase photosensitivity and are best diffused or applied to the skin with limited sun exposure. Diluting essential oils in a carrier oil base reduces their photosensitivity effects. Please check your blends and become familiar with the ones that contain oils that increase photosensitivity. The individual oils that may cause photosensitivity include:

- **Angelica** (*Angelica archangelica*)
- **Bergamot** (*Citrus bergamia*)
- **Grapefruit** (*Citrus paradisi*)
- **Lemon** (*Citrus limon*)
- **Lime** (*Citrus aurantifolia*)
- **Orange** (*Citrus aurantium*)
- **Petitgrain** (*Citrus aurantium*)
- **Rue** (*Ruta graveolens*)

In general, the best location to apply essential oils when combining with astrological influences is the associated acupuncture point (described in a later chapter). You can also apply the diluted blend to the back of the neck, the face, outer ear, and spinal column (this allows the essential oil to cross the blood-brain barrier and calm the central nervous system.) Rotating the application sites reduces the risk of skin irritation with long-term use. Each planetary and sign blend has application recommendations and uses discussed in detail throughout this book.

Cautions When Using Essential Oils

Never apply essential oils near your eyes or inside your ear canals. If an essential oil gets too close to the eye and causes irritation, apply vegetable oil around the orb (the bony socket surrounding the eye), and blink it into your eye, if needed, to dilute the essential oil. If an essential oil is too close to your ear canal, dip a Q-tip in vegetable oil and gently apply it to the outer edge of your ear canal, allowing it to drip inside the ear. Rinsing your eyes or ear canals with water will only increase the irritation.

Remember to dilute an essential oil with vegetable oil and do not attempt to rinse it off first with water. You can safely wash the essential oils off your hands by using a liberal amount of soap before rinsing your hands with water. You can wash the essential oils off other areas (not the eyes and ears) by diluting with carrier oil, then washing with soap, then applying carrier oil again.

Therapeutic-grade essential oils lose their healing properties when heated to above 120 degrees Fahrenheit. So avoid storing your oils in direct sunlight, in your car during the summer, or near the stove, etc. Storing your essential oils in a cool and dark location will help preserve their healing potential. Blends mixed with carrier oil can become rancid after a few years of storage. Pure oils, if stored properly, will last for years.

All Essential Oils Are Not Created Equal

There are three grades of essential oils: food grade, perfume grade, and therapeutic grade. Food-grade and perfume-grade oils use the cheapest manufacturing methods available. Chemicals used in the food-grade and perfume-grade manufacturing processes include pesticides and fertilizers applied during the plants' growing stages as well as toxic solvents used for extracting their oils. Diluted food-grade oils contain only a small percentage of the essential oil to keep costs down and often contain preservatives. We do not recommend these oils for internal use, and some can be harmful when ingested.

Therapeutic-grade essential oils vary in quality and fragrance from one manufacturer to another. Conventionally grown, organic, and wild-harvested plants used to make therapeutic-grade essential oils all differ in their aromas and healing properties, based on farming practices and geographical location. Most therapeutic-grade essential oil manufacturers use a steam distillation extraction process, the preferred method, but others use chemical solvents to increase yields. In some cases, lower quality or less expensive therapeutic-grade essential oils can lower your electrical frequency and cause unwanted side effects.

The Planetary and Sign Essential Oil Blends

Michelle Meramour carefully formulated the planetary (meridian balancing) and sign (organ supporting) essential oil blends. She used her Meramour's Body-Feedback muscle testing techniques to make sure they corrected meridian and organ imbalances and supported a person's healing process on all levels. In 2009, Michelle began incorporating essential oil blends into her treatments, and she categorized their attributes based on Chinese medical theory and the various blends' healing and chemical properties. Michelle then confirmed the accuracy of her classifications over the next five years by testing them on an average of fifty clients per week totaling over 12,000 treatments. This knowledge base and years of experience along with her intuition guided her to formulate the unique blends for the planets and signs.

The planetary blends consist of three essential oils, an odd or yang number that represents the active and changing nature of both the planets and the meridians. A balanced meridian system supports physical health and emotional resiliency. Intentionally working with your planetary aspects to the Sun and Moon in your birth chart can soften challenging themes in your life while enhancing your natural strengths.

The sign blends consist of four essential oils, an even or yin number that represents a solid foundation, stability, and predictability. The sign blends relate to the signs of the zodiac and our organ systems. When worked with consciously, the sign blends foster increased self-awareness, healthy relationships, and emotional stability.

Essential oil substitutions for the planetary and sign blends included in this book cover the basic safety precautions for high blood pressure and pregnancy. If you have a serious medical condition, please consult your physician and licensed healthcare providers before using essential oils. At times, certain oils may become unavailable because they come from nature with a limited supply. Throughout this book, Michelle recommends specific application methods, cautions, and substitutions by the blend. Always remember to check with your essential oil manufacturer for acceptable uses and application methods.

Allie's Experience with Astrology Blends

In the introduction, we described Allie's journey toward higher vibrational living. Once she began using the astrology blends, Allie noticed that they worked better with her body's chemistry than other oils, and the aroma was surprisingly appealing to people she encountered. Allie also found the effects of these essential oil blends lasted longer, which allowed her to reapply them less often while feeling the full benefits.

Archetypes of the Sun and Moon

*What I know for sure: There is no greater gift
you can give or receive than to honor your calling.
It's why you were born. And how you become most truly alive.*

—Oprah Winfrey

The Sun and Moon in your birth chart are particularly foundational to who you are. The Sun relates to your core identity and personality, and the Moon relates to your emotional nature and the ways that you deal with your body, health, and emotions. By understanding your sun and moon signs and their interactions with other planets in your birth chart, you gain insight into who you are, your core strengths and weaknesses, as well as core themes in your life. These luminaries and their aspects to the other planets are the focus of this book since they are the cornerstones of the natal birth chart and of your identity.

The signs of the Western astrology zodiac trace the path of the Sun across the year and reflect the energies of the different seasonal cycles. Your birth chart both shows where the Sun is in the seasonal cycle (by the sign that it is in). Where the Sun, Moon, and planets are located in the chart (by house placements) is based on the time of day when you were born.

The planets reflect core archetypes that relate to aspects of who you are. The energies of the planets correspond to the sign and house of your birth chart in which they reside as well as to which aspects they have with other planets in your chart. Together these shape how the planetary archetypes manifest in your life and personality. Later on in this section, you will find descriptions of the key archetypes of the planets and signs, as well as the meanings of their house placements, to guide you as to how they weave together.

In Chinese medicine, eight special vessels, which are different from the meridians, become active before birth. Two of them, the governing and conception vessels, strongly influence your physical and emotional development. These two special vessels carry your DNA as well as your core strengths and weaknesses in this lifetime. Your sun sign corresponds with the governing vessel, which controls the yang meridians and more masculine functions of the body (warming, outward, and active functions). Your moon sign corresponds with the conception vessel, which controls the yin meridians and more feminine functions of the body (the cooling, internal, and restorative functions).

Finding Your Own Path to Higher Vibrational Living

Identifying Your Sun and Moon Signs in Your Birth Chart

In this section, you will learn how to use your birth chart to understand the core themes of your sun and moon signs. You will also learn how to use the astrology blends to support moving into higher vibrational living through alignment with your true self.

You can obtain your natal chart information two different ways. You can work with a professional astrologer or look up your birth chart on the internet, and there are advantages to both. You will need your birth time as well as your birth date and place. If you do not know your birth time, you can contact the town or city hall of your birthplace and request it. While hospitals do not keep birth records long-term, city halls usually keep permanent records.

It would be helpful to work with a professional astrologer if you are unsure of your exact birth time, if the free charts online do not resonate with how you see yourself, or you are finding it difficult to work with the free software programs available online. Also, if you are looking for a more in-depth understanding of your birth chart with opportunities to ask questions and address particular issues, then a professional astrologer is a good choice. A professional astrologer can also provide insights about how the current planetary energies (transits) are coming into play in your chart and in your life. You can use the information about your current astrological influences with the upcoming planetary and sign blends also. When choosing an astrologer to work with, please check for reviews and testimonials online or from other people before deciding on one.

Free astrology chart programs are available on the internet from a variety of websites, which enable you to view your chart, and some allow you to print it. In addition to obtaining your birth chart, these websites usually provide basic astrology education, again for free, and more advanced information or computer-generated readings for a charge or a subscription fee. However, these reports are generic in nature and will not be able to provide the depth of information about you and your unique strengths and weaknesses that you would gain from a professional astrologer. When using an online astrology site as with any website, you should check for reviews from other users and check a few before deciding on one that will work for you.

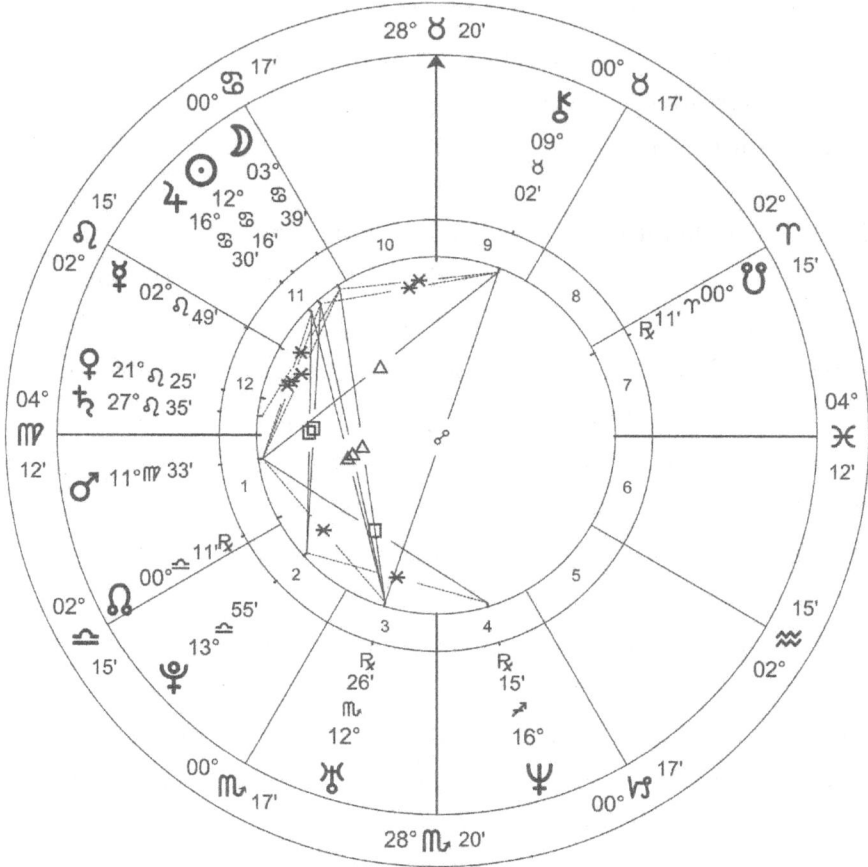

Allie's Birth Chart

The Sun Archetype: Your True Essence

The Sun is central in your birth chart and reflects your core identity and the uniqueness of who you are. Just as the Sun is at the center of our solar system and is the source of light and life for our planet, the sun sign in your birth chart shows the light and essence of who you are and how you can be in alignment with your true self. The Sun shows your core personality traits and strengths and weaknesses.

Once you have obtained your birth chart, locate your sun sign and see if you connect with the basic meaning of this sign as described below. When you support the energy of who you are, raise your vibration, and deepen your self-awareness, you can live out the best qualities of this sun sign. You will soon see if you have difficult or supportive aspects to your Sun in your chart. If you have challenging aspects, it may be hard to feel grounded in who you are and to live up to your full potential. The aspects are explained below; usually, the squares and oppositions are the most challenging aspects. Once you work these challenges consciously and use the astrology oil blends to support you in aligning with your true self, these challenging aspects can become strengths rather than blocks to self-expression. If you have supportive aspects, those other planetary energies are helping you more easily access the essence of who you are.

In later chapters, you will find more in-depth descriptions of the energies of each planet as well as the signs of the zodiac.

Key Phrases for Each Sun Sign of the Zodiac

ARIES SUN:
Enjoys taking action and learning through experience.

TAURUS SUN:
Values security and consistency and is grounded.

GEMINI SUN:
Loves to learn, to communicate, and to connect with others.

CANCER SUN:
Is nurturing, caring, and emotionally sensitive.

LEO SUN:

Values self-expression, creativity, and living from the heart.
The Sun is the ruler of Leo and is especially strong in this sign.

VIRGO SUN:

Seeks self-improvement and to be of service to others.

LIBRA SUN:

Values one-on-one relationships and understands different
perspectives.

SCORPIO SUN:

Is intense and has strong views about life.

SAGITTARIUS SUN:

Enjoys adventure, exploration, and formulating personal beliefs.

CAPRICORN SUN:

Values being responsible, disciplined, and achieving goals.

AQUARIUS SUN:

Cares about social issues and enjoys being in groups.

PISCES SUN:

Values dreams and wants to be of service to something larger
than the self.

House Placement

Once you have determined your sun sign, look to see which segment or house your Sun resides in by looking at the numbers in the inner wheel of your natal chart. These twelve segments of the chart show which area of life is a key focus for you. Following are the meanings of each of the houses in the natal chart.

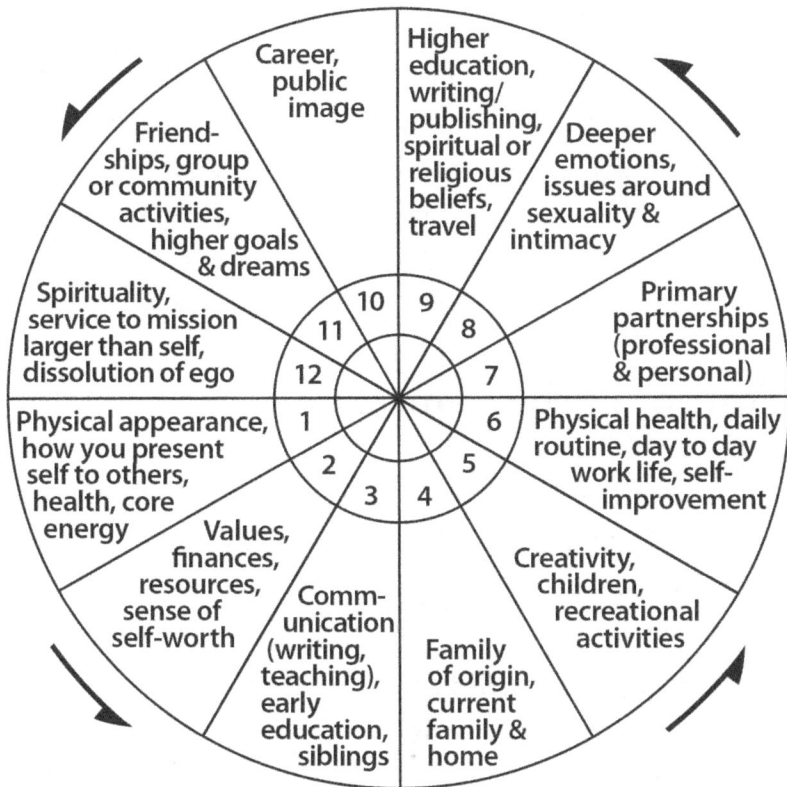

Key Words for Houses

Aspects

After finding your Sun's house placement, examine what aspects your Sun has by looking at the lines connecting your Sun to other planets in your chart. These connections with the other planets add more meaning to the themes that may be important in your life and to your unique gifts or challenges.

The connections between the Sun and other planets may be supportive or challenging. By looking at the specific aspects to your Sun, you gain more understanding of your strengths as well as areas of vulnerability or difficulty. As you gain awareness of these energies that are part of who you are and work to raise your vibrational level, you can access the gifts of these patterns rather than getting caught in the challenges they may represent.

Meanings of the Planetary Aspects

Following are the key symbols for the aspects and their meanings. When working with planetary aspects to the Sun or Moon, the planet should be within ten degrees of the Sun or Moon.

CONJUNCTION: This aspect occurs when a planet is next to the Sun or Moon in the natal chart and is within ten degrees of either luminary. (Conjunctions with other planets are when two planets are within 5 degrees of each other.) A conjunction with the Sun or Moon indicates that the energy of the other planet will be a strong influence in your life. This influence can be either supportive or challenging depending on how you work with it. When two other planets are conjunct, their energies blend together.

✳ **SEXTILE:** A sextile is when two planets are approximately sixty degrees apart. This supportive aspect adds positive energy from the other planet to the energy of your Sun or Moon and indicates strengths or gifts that are a conscious part of your identity. A sextile between two other planets indicates that these parts of yourself are integrated and supportive of each other.

☐ **SQUARE:** A square is when two planets are approximately ninety degrees apart. This is one of the more challenging aspects in the natal chart. It shows an inner conflict or part of your identity that may be hard for you to integrate, especially if it is a square between a planet and the Sun or Moon. As you learn more about this planet's energy and work with the astrology blends, you can shift this aspect into being an area of strength in your life and develop more insight about yourself. If it is a square between two other planets, these facets of your personality may be in conflict or tension with each other.

△ **TRINE:** A trine is when two planets are approximately 120 degrees apart. The trine is a supportive aspect and represents a gift or strength that you have naturally. You may take this part of yourself for granted, but others see and appreciate this aspect of who you are.

☍ **OPPOSITION:** An opposition is when two planets are approximately 180 degrees apart. This challenging aspect occurs when another planet is opposite your Sun or Moon, or when two planets are opposite each other. When a planet is in opposition with the Sun or Moon, the opposing planet represents a strong part of who you are, but you may have difficulty fully accepting or integrating this quality in yourself. You may tend to project this trait on to others, while not always understanding how it is part of you.

If you have *beneficial* aspects to the Sun in your birth chart, you will likely feel self-confident and at ease in expressing yourself. You are also apt to have good vitality and strong energy. You will manifest the energy of the sign in which your Sun resides with ease and live out the highest qualities of that sign.

If you have *challenging* aspects to the Sun in your birth chart, you may struggle to have a clear sense of yourself, or you may feel blocked in living out the truth or light of who you are. With several challenging aspects, you may find yourself struggling with low energy, and difficulties with self-confidence and self-expression, as well as possible constitutional health issues related to the sign the Sun is in. You may also feel insecure in how you interact with others and may struggle to manifest your goals.

The natal Sun (along with Saturn) also reflects the nature of our relationships with our fathers. Beneficial aspects to the Sun can indicate a positive relationship with your father, suggesting that you experienced him as supportive of you. With challenging aspects to the Sun, you may have found it difficult to relate to your father or felt that the relationship was often strained or conflictual. This difficult relationship may have a significant impact on your underlying sense of confidence and may result in feelings of insecurity and inadequacy.

Challenging Aspects to the Sun

The challenging aspects to the Sun are the ones that are most likely the source of emotional or physical difficulties in your life. Following is a description of how these aspects might manifest. It is important to integrate the energies of the signs that the Sun and challenging planet reside in as well as the energy of the aspect.

CONJUNCTIONS

The archetypal energy of the planet may be overshadowed, especially when in aspect to the Sun. When a planet is near the Sun, it becomes invisible and is "under the beams of the Sun." This may weaken that planet's energy, and the energy of the planet will be merged with that of the Sun.

SUN/MERCURY:

This aspect may manifest in a blending of your thoughts and sense of self. At times, this may indicate some difficulties in self-expression due to the way that Mercury is merged with the Sun.

SUN/VENUS:

You value relationships and may have difficulty having a clear sense of yourself apart from your significant relationships. You may grow and evolve through your relationship experiences.

SUN/MARS:

You live out who you are through your actions. You may also tend, at times, to be in conflict with yourself and channel the Mars energy inward.

SUN/JUPITER:

You have self-confidence and enjoy expressing yourself. You may at times be overly idealistic or have an inflated sense of self.

SUN/SATURN:

You may have had difficulties in your relationship with your father in childhood and have a tendency to be self-critical. You may not feel easily understood by others but, if you work with this aspect consciously, you have the potential to develop a strong sense of self and come to honor your own inner authority.

SUN/URANUS:

You are likely to have the energy of a reformer or rebel. You value independence and authenticity and may have difficulties with authorities or with situations in which you see injustice or the abuse of power. If not worked consciously, this aspect can lead to a lack of a clear sense of self and possible egotistical traits.

SUN/NEPTUNE:

This aspect is an indicator of sensitivity, compassion, and intuitive gifts. In childhood, this can mean difficulties in separating your sense of self from those around you. This may manifest in adulthood as difficulties with boundaries and a tendency to adapt to those around you, leading to some confusion about your sense of self.

SUN/PLUTO:

This combination indicates a depth, intensity, and more introverted sense of self. You may be a markedly private person and sensitive to any experiences of intrusion or abuse. You have a strong will and inner power.

SQUARES

When a planet is squaring the Sun, it conflicts with the energy of the Sun. This aspect may reflect an inner conflict that needs to be resolved in order to have a more integrated sense of self. Note that Mercury and Venus are never far enough from the Sun to be in this aspect.

SUN/MARS:

You may have difficulties in how you act or assert yourself. You may alternate between holding yourself back and then becoming angry or overly assertive.

SUN/JUPITER:

You may have an inflated sense of self or a have difficulties with self-confidence. To balance this, you will need to examine your beliefs and high expectations in order to see yourself more clearly and have reasonable goals.

SUN/SATURN:

This aspect is likely to manifest in early issues around feelings of being misunderstood, leading to a tendency to be self-critical or to doubt yourself. When worked through, this combination can lead to inner strength and to finding your own inner authority.

SUN/URANUS:

You may experience a conflict between your desire for change and your need for security. You may vacillate between wanting to be unconventional and unique and wanting to fit in and be more "part of the crowd."

SUN/NEPTUNE:

You may have a high level of sensitivity and a tendency to want to escape or numb yourself in times of stress. You will need to learn to manage your sensitivity, have clear boundaries, and trust your intuitive nature.

SUN/PLUTO:

You may feel in conflict with your intensity and may have a tendency to become depressed or to hold yourself back. You may also engage in power struggles with others as a way of compensating for feelings of powerlessness.

OPPOSITIONS

When a planet is opposite the Sun, you may tend to disown this part of yourself and see it in others or experience it through a relationship. The challenge is to integrate this as an aspect of yourself. Oppositions with the outermost planets are the most challenging. Note that it is not possible to have an opposition between the Sun and Mercury or Venus due to the closeness of their orbits with the Sun.

SUN/MARS:

You may tend to get into conflicts with others but not see yourself as an aggressive person. As you own your own anger and assertive nature, you will be able to be more in balance with this energy. This then manifests as being assertive and active rather than tending to get into conflicts with others.

SUN/JUPITER:

You may be drawn to others with whom you relate as mentors or teachers. It is important to honor your own faith, beliefs, and gifts as a teacher or guide to others.

SUN/SATURN:

You may tend to get into relationships with others who are either critical or controlling of you, exacerbating your lack of self-esteem. As you honor your own inner strength, you will be more able to set clear boundaries with others and engage in more balanced relationships.

SUN/URANUS:

You are attracted to people that you see as creative, unconventional, reformers or pioneers. It is important to honor your own uniqueness, independence, and unconventional nature.

SUN/NEPTUNE:

You may tend to be compassionate and hold high ideals, but you may often project your own vulnerabilities or strengths on to others, not seeing them or yourself clearly. It is important to be compassionate with yourself and to honor both your strengths and your weaknesses.

SUN/PLUTO:

You may tend to get into power struggles with others, perceiving others as being abusive or domineering with you. It is important to honor your own intensity and power which then allows you to relate to others in a more mutual way.

Supportive Aspects to the Sun

SEXTILES AND TRINES

At times, conjunctions may be supportive aspects to the Sun, depending on how you work with the blending of the energy of the Sun with that particular planet. However, the most supportive aspects are the sextiles and trines. The sextiles indicate gifts or strengths that you may be well aware of and working consciously, while the trines are usually more intrinsic aspects of who you are. Following are some of the ways that planets that are in these beneficial aspects with the Sun may manifest in your life.

SUN/MARS:

You are likely to have a good energy level and the ability to take action based on who you are and what is important to you.

SUN/JUPITER:

You are likely to have a strong sense of self-confidence and a sense of optimism about life. You have faith that things will work out even when in challenging circumstances.

SUN/SATURN:

You have a strong sense of self, clear boundaries, and are able to stay focused on what is important to you.

SUN/URANUS:

You are comfortable with being different and following your own instincts. You are apt to be creative and innovative in how you approach life. You also value authenticity and fairness in interactions with others.

SUN/NEPTUNE:

You are likely to be compassionate, sensitive, and caring. You may love music, film, art, or photography and have creative gifts. You may also be spiritual or have a strong desire to be of service in the world.

SUN/PLUTO:

You have a depth and intensity with regard to who you are and may have a strong drive to pursue what is important to you. You have inner strength and an ability to handle stress and crises with resiliency.

Examples of Sun Signs and Their Aspects

To aid in understanding how these aspects manifest in real life, we will explore the primary aspects to the Sun and Moon in Allie's chart as well as in the charts of Oprah Winfrey and Deepak Chopra.

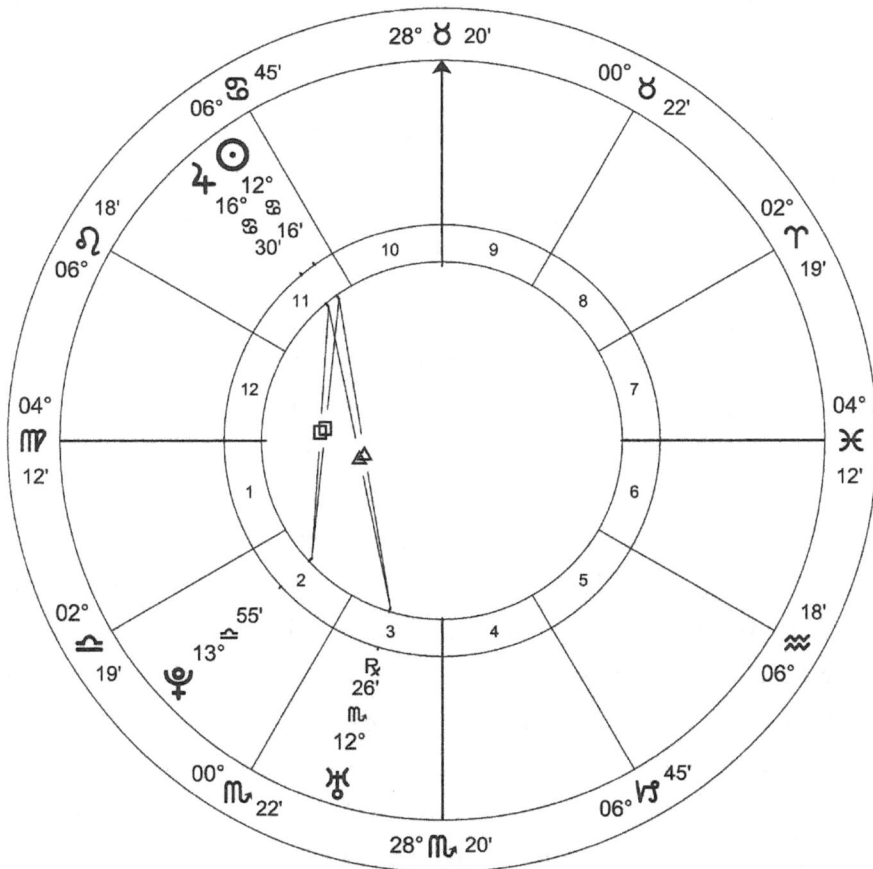

Allie's Chart with Sun Aspects

Allie's Sun Sign and House Placement: In Allie's chart, her sun sign is in Cancer and is in the eleventh house. These indicate that she is a caring, nurturing, and emotionally sensitive person who enjoys working in group situations and investing her energy in her goals.

Allie's Aspects to the Sun: Note that, in Allie's chart, Jupiter is next to her Sun indicating that she is likely to have a sense of self-confidence and strong ideals. Her Sun is also in a square with Pluto, meaning that she is intense, driven, and prone to burn-out. This configuration could also indicate a challenging relationship with her father. This is a difficult aspect and one that would be important for her to deal with consciously and to support with essential oils. This would help her work the challenging aspect at a high vibrational level. Allie's Sun is also in a trine with Uranus, which shows that she enjoys being creative and working independently and may be frustrated in situations that do not allow her the full expression of her gifts (such as a corporate environment).

In Chinese medicine, the sign of Cancer corresponds to the processing of sugar and carbohydrates along with converting food into energy and blood. With Allie's Sun and Moon and the planet Jupiter in the sign of Cancer, she experiences increased inflammation and hormonal imbalances when she consumes sugar in her diet. Allie's blood sugar levels become unstable after high carbohydrate meals, which causes her to feel tired after eating. The Pluto square relates to the adrenals and the endocrine system in Chinese medicine, and Allie has experienced adrenal fatigue and hormonal imbalances due to stress and excessive sugar. The Uranus trine enhances her physical health and her work as a yoga instructor in that it supports her connective tissue and increases her flexibility.

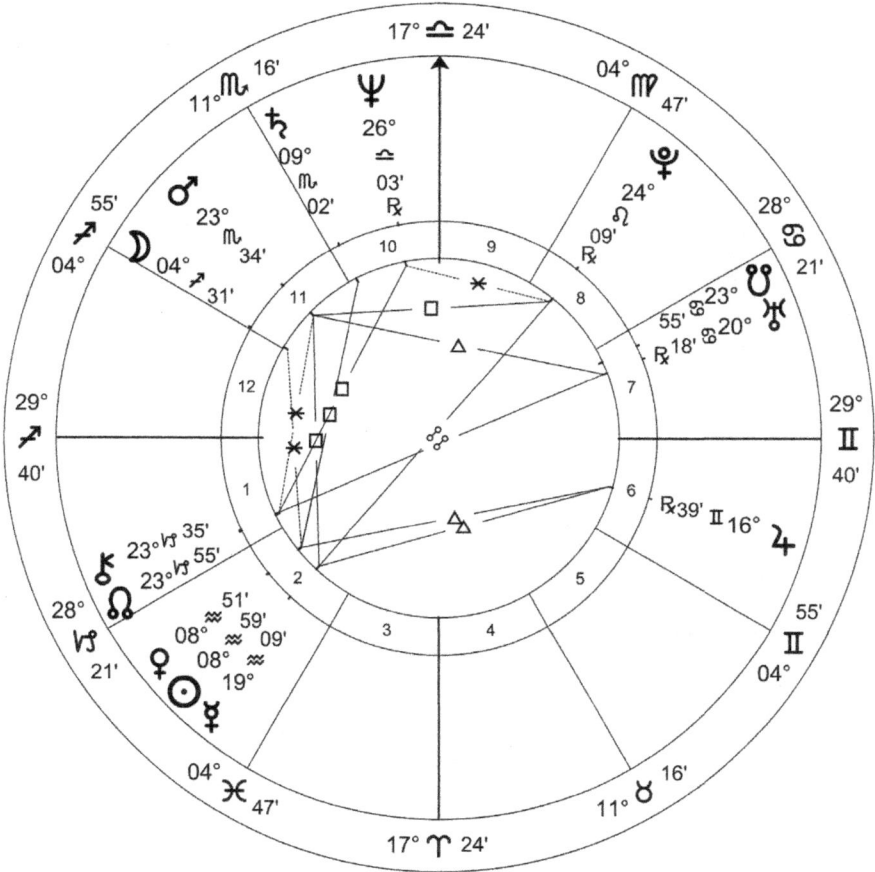

Oprah Winfrey's Natal Chart

Oprah's Sun Sign and House Placement: In her birth chart, Oprah's sun sign is in Aquarius in the second house. Her Sun in Aquarius indicates strong concerns about social issues and her effectiveness in relating with a diversity of people. With her Sun in the second house, Oprah exhibits strong values, is concerned about having financial security, and may also have issues with her self-esteem.

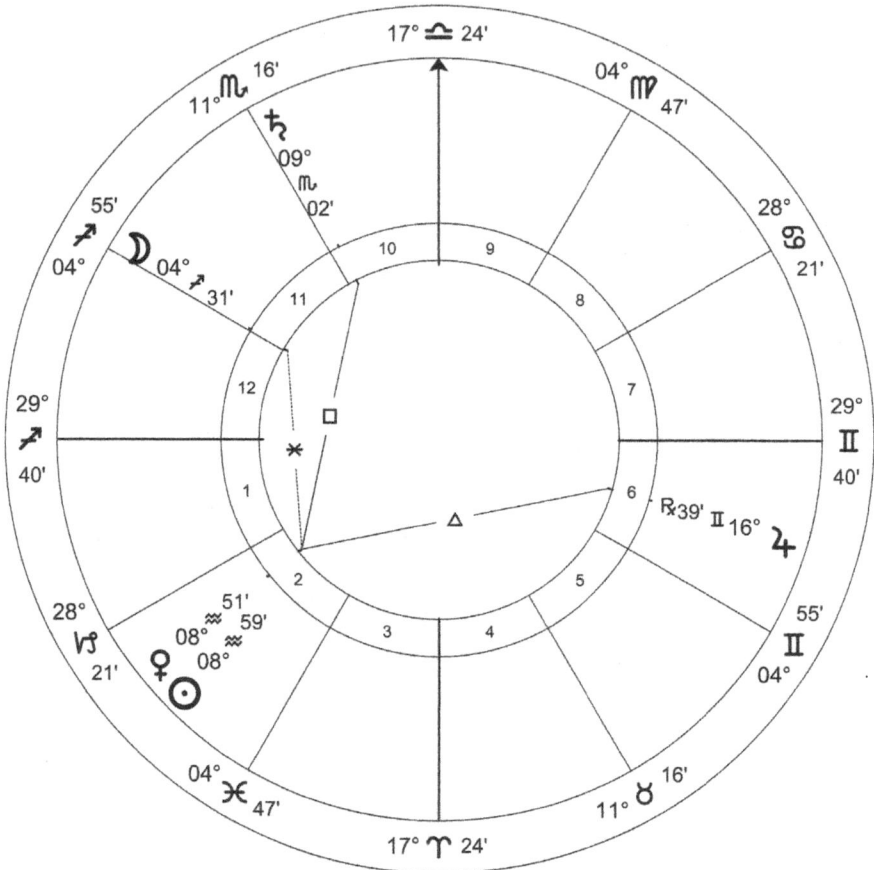

Oprah Winfrey's Chart with Sun Aspects

Oprah's Aspects to the Sun: Oprah's Sun is next to Venus indicating that she strongly values relationships and that her capacity to relate well with others is a core part of her identity. With her Sun in a supportive aspect (sextile) with the Moon, her sense of herself and her emotional nature are not in conflict with each other but tend to be integrated and mutually supportive. Oprah's Sun also has a supportive aspect (trine) with Jupiter, which gives her a sense of confidence and an optimistic and outgoing nature. This can indicate that she experienced her father as supportive of her. Her Sun has a challenging aspect (square) with Saturn. This can indicate periods of self-doubt or the experience of growing up not feeling understood or affirmed by other authority figures in her life. However, as she works with this aspect, it can support her in having a strong sense of self and inner strength.

In Chinese medicine, the sign of Aquarius relates to the gallbladder organ and is responsible for the digestion of fats. Oprah's very close conjunction with Venus influences sugar and carbohydrate processing that affects both the nervous system (Venus as an evening star) and metabolism (Venus as a morning star). This combination can create a challenge when digesting fats and carbohydrates in the same meal and results in higher blood sugar levels and increased fat storage within the cells.

The two planets in aspect to Oprah's natal Sun, Saturn and Jupiter, correspond with the lymph system and the pituitary brain connection that controls all hormones in the body. Since hormones are made from healthy fats, Oprah's endocrine system and hormonal balance are directly impacted by the quality of fats in her diet, and she would feel best if she consumed primarily Omega 3 fats from fish, olive oil, and avocados. The square from Saturn forces Oprah to restrict her carbohydrate intake or she will retain fluids in the lymph system, and to limit the consumption of unhealthy fats or she will store them because her body cannot effectively use them. The trine from Jupiter provides high energy levels, which is best used for physical activity or the high energy will turn to stress hormones and increase the storage of fat around the abdomen.

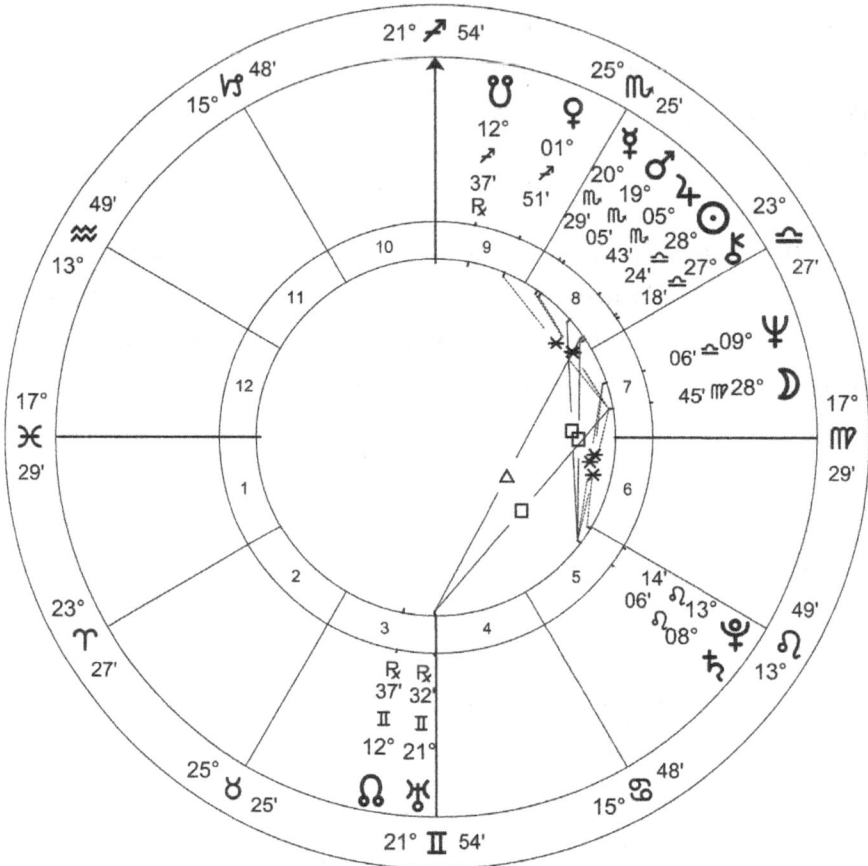

Deepak Chopra's Natal Chart

Deepak's Sun Sign and House Placement: Deepak's Sun, in his birth chart, is in Libra, indicating that he values harmony and balance. Being in the eighth house, he may be focused on understanding himself and others at a deep level and more introverted than extroverted.

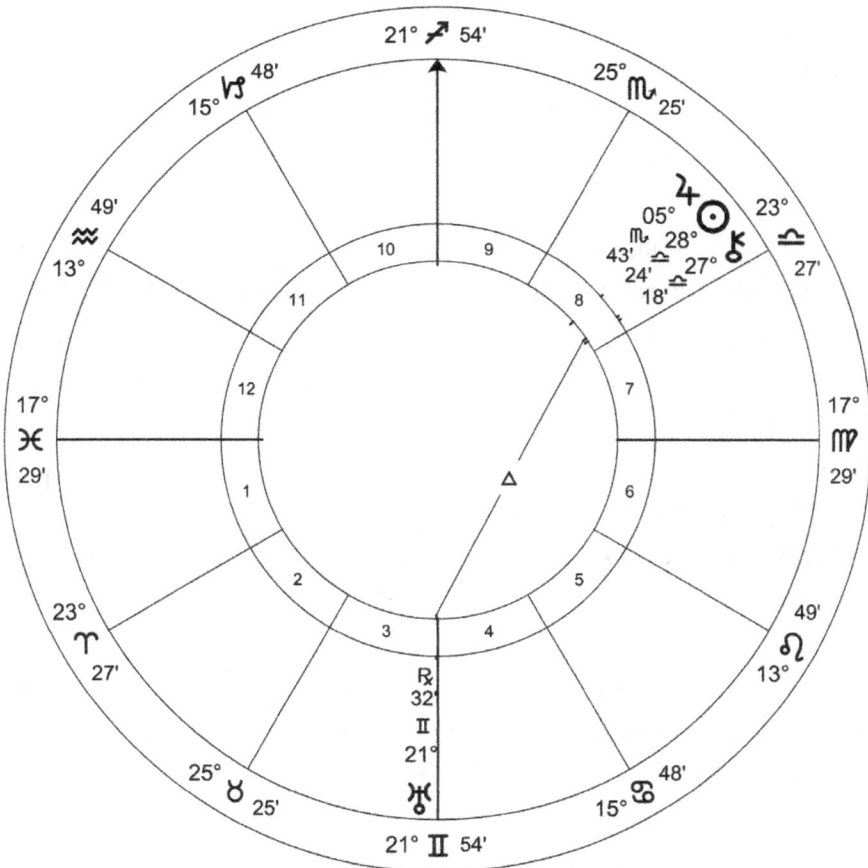

Deepak Chopra's Chart with Sun Aspects

Deepak's Aspects to the Sun: Deepak's Sun is next to Jupiter, reflecting a strong faith and optimistic approach to life. It also indicates having the gifts of a teacher. With Chiron next to his Sun, Deepak may have to work through some issues around his sense of his own identity and his understanding of healing. This aspect also shows his natural abilities as a healer as he does his own inner work and seeks to understand others as an integration of mind, body, and spirit. With his Sun in a supportive aspect to Uranus (trine), he is creative, innovative, and unconventional in his approach to life.

In Chinese medicine, the sign of Libra relates to the bladder organ, which requires healthy hormones and nerve conduction to function properly. Increased inflammation and stress negatively impact bladder function.

The very close conjunction with Chiron in the sign of Libra further intensifies the relationship with bladder function in Chinese medicine. The small intestine meridian works closely with the bladder by influencing the hypothalamus master gland in the brain. This combination gives Deepak a deep understanding of how thoughts influence the nervous system. Deepak's books and teachings often include the message that how you choose to view life directly impacts physical and emotional health through conscious thought patterns.

Deepak's Sun conjunction with Jupiter corresponds with the pericardium meridian in Chinese medicine. The pericardium meridian influences the pituitary and controls all hormones in the body. Mental health and emotional health together depend on balanced hormones, including the stress hormone cortisol. This combined conjunction of Chiron and Jupiter with Deepak's natal Sun would cause him to be keenly aware of how thoughts and emotions affect his health and vitality. Both of these meridians influence the digestive process, and the quality of foods eaten will directly impact mental and emotional health.

The planet Uranus creates a trine with Deepak's natal Sun and Chiron. Uranus corresponds with the gallbladder meridian and the digestion of healthy fats. The brain and all hormones depend on the digestion of healthy fats. The Uranus trine strengthens Deepak's digestion. It also aids his ability to regenerate the brain and nervous system as he consumes healthy fats in his diet.

The Natal Sun Sign and the Governing Vessel

The energy of the Sun in your birth chart corresponds with the governing vessel in traditional Chinese medicine. The governing vessel, known as the "Sea of Yang Channels," includes the brain and spinal cord and controls the spinal nerves and the cerebrospinal fluid. The governing vessel relates to the hypothalamus gland, which gathers and filters information from the nervous system as you experience the world. The governing vessel has the strongest influence on how you perceive the world, your personality, and your mental capacity. Your will to persevere, your ability to take action, and your connection to your higher-self are all accessed through the governing vessel.

In traditional Chinese medicine, conception occurs when the mother's and father's essence meet; thus, the governing and conception vessels form first. Today this is recognized as the blending of the parents' DNA, which occurs when the sperm and egg meet. As the sperm enters the egg, the first cells divide and create the right and left sides of the body. The governing vessel controls the yang, the masculine characteristics, and the right side of the body. The conception vessel controls the yin, the feminine characteristics, and the left side of the body. The governing vessel provides the spark of life needed to create a new being. This spark of life, or flame, is yang and represents the ancestral lineage that forms the masculine functions expressed through the governing vessel.

This spark of life created by the governing vessel at conception is with you for your entire life. This inner light can illuminate your life path and your destiny by governing your thoughts, which become your actions. When your actions align with your higher vibrational self, your life direction becomes clear, and your decisions have integrity.

Working with the energy of your natal Sun through the governing vessel can provide clarity of thought for well-executed plans and the drive needed for action. The Natal Sun Luminary Blend can help integrate your planetary aspects with your sense of self. By combining the Natal Sun Luminary Blend with a *challenging* planetary aspect blend, you can gain the wisdom born from working through difficult situations. By combining the Natal Sun Luminary Blend with a *beneficial* planetary blend, your natural talents and abilities will shine through.

Allie's natal Sun is in the sign of Cancer with a square (challenging aspect) to the planet Pluto, and a trine (beneficial aspect) to the planet Uranus. When Allie finds herself in power struggles or controlling situations, she can combine the Natal Sun Luminary Blend with the Pluto Planetary Blend to help her consciously make decisions that support transformation. When Allie is working independently or engaged in projects involving new concepts, social justice, or improving the lives of others, she can combine the Natal Sun Luminary Blend with the Uranus Planetary Blend to support her generation of new ideas, her connection with society, and her follow-through to achieve her goals.

The Harmonizing Essence of the Natal Sun Luminary Blend

The Natal Sun Luminary Blend (also known as the Du/Governing Vessel Meridian Balancing Blend), consists of 50% sacred frankincense (*Boswellia sacra*), 25% sandalwood (*Santalum album*), and 25% blue spruce (*Picea pungens*). Sacred frankincense comes from the Oman region in the Middle East, and many believe it to be the type of frankincense brought to the birth of Jesus. Other types of frankincense are mainly found in Africa and the Middle

East. Ancient cultures believed that frankincense carried the energy and healing light of the Sun.

Ancient cultures considered sandalwood to be sacred and incorporated it at birth and death ceremonies to aid the soul in passing between the worlds. In the Natal Sun Luminary Blend, sandalwood helps the spirit to feel at home in the physical body and safe in the immediate environment. Both are functions of the hypothalamus.

In Chinese medicine today, frankincense resin is commonly used in herbal formulas as *ru xiang*. *Ru xiang* regulates blood flow, relaxes the muscles, alleviates, pain, and generates flesh. *Ru xiang* is most often combined with *mo yao*, the resin of myrrh, which is a key ingredient in the Natal Moon Luminary Blend. Together frankincense and myrrh resin are commonly used in Chinese medicine for pain from trauma or any obstruction affecting the meridian system.

Many Native American Indians consider spruce trees to be sacred today. They believe these trees provide protection and communication from the heavens. The spruce trees in areas of Canada and the northern United States reach up to touch the aurora borealis, or northern lights, a beautiful display caused when high-energy solar particles from the Sun penetrate the Earth's magnetic shield, colliding with the atoms in the atmosphere. This collision causes the excited atoms to give off energy in the form of multicolored light. Blue spruce blends best with the sacred frankincense.

If sacred frankincense or blue spruce is unavailable, then substituting with black spruce (*picea mariana*) and regular frankincense (*boswellia carterii*) is best. Black spruce combines better with regular frankincense. Blue spruce combines better with sacred frankincense.

The essential oils that make up the Natal Sun Luminary Blend come from trees and are high in sesquiterpenes, which raise consciousness and activate the pineal gland. In astrology, the Sun relates to the pineal gland and higher states of consciousness. Ongoing exposure to the energy of sunlight at dawn or sunset also activates the pineal gland.

How to Use the Natal Sun Luminary Blend

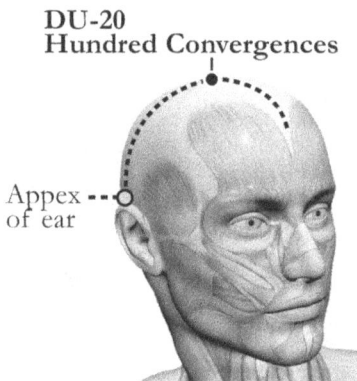

DU-20
Hundred Convergences

Appex
of ear

The governing vessel has two important acupuncture points that support the energy of the natal Sun. Hundred Convergences, also known as *Bai Hui*, Governing Vessel 20, GV-20, or DU-20, is found at the vertex of the head in line with the apex of the ears. This becomes the highest point in the body when standing straight with good posture. In Chinese, the character for *Bai* stands for "many," and this point is known as the meeting point of a hundred spirits or the meeting point of many meridians. When this acupuncture point needs attention, it becomes tender to the touch, which makes it easier to find.

Applying a drop of the Natal Sun Luminary Blend on Hundred Convergences on the top of the head can help strengthen your connection to Spirit, your higher self, God, or your Creator. Energizing this acupuncture point with the Natal Sun Luminary Blend and the following affirmations promotes alignment to your eternal energy source as represented by your natal Sun. If you meditate or pray, try using this blend on the top of the head to call upon your hundred spirit guides and guardian angels. Visualize light coming from the Sun and filling your brain and spinal column with golden, healing light and love.

Life Gate, also known as *Ming Men*, Governing Vessel 4, GV-4, or DU-4, is found on the lower back, just below the second lumbar vertebra and on the spine. When standing, you can find this point by first resting your hands on the highest point of the hipbone on your back. Then follow this level to the spine and move up an inch to find your Life Gate point. Chinese medicine associates this point with both the ancestral *qi* acquired from your parents as well as the life force passed on to future generations.

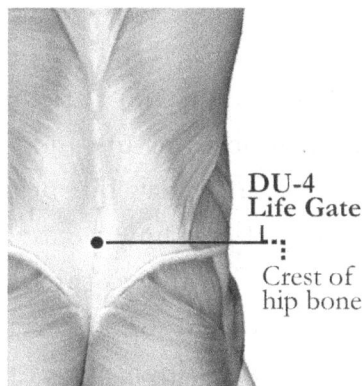

DU-4
Life Gate

Crest of
hip bone

Applying a few drops, in a clockwise motion, of the Natal Sun Luminary Blend with a challenging planetary aspect blend to Life Gate can help you learn and grow from difficult situations associated with your father or other authority figures. Combining the Natal Sun Luminary Blend with beneficial planetary aspects can energize your life force and ignite your passions. Apply your oils with intention and combine the application with an affirmation.

| *Natal Sun Luminary Affirmations:* | I am secure in who I am.

I am filled with light and life.

I live out who I am in the world. |

The Moon Archetype:
Your Emotional Nature

The Moon in the sky dances with the Sun and moves through cycles of light and dark. In our birth charts, the Moon reveals our emotional nature and how we experience being in our bodies. As the Sun shows our personalities and essential identities, the Moon reflects how we experience life in emotional and physical ways. In that it goes through its cycle of waxing and waning each month, the Moon also relates to the cycles in our lives. Every month, the Moon moves through a cycle of being in darkness, birthing into light, growing, evolving, coming into fullness, then gradually fading and disappearing once again. In this way, the Moon is showing us how our lives are a constant cycle of change, of beginnings, completions, and transitions and that we, like everything on Earth, move through a process of life/death/rebirth. The Moon also strongly affects the cycles of plants and animals as well as controlling the tides of the larger bodies of water.

Historically, before modern birth control and wide use of artificial light, menstruating women were in tune with the energy of the Moon. They ovulated at the time of the full Moon and menstruated at the time of the new Moon. Today, because of birth control, endocrine disorders, and light pollution, most women are no longer naturally synchronized to the Moon. Today, for both men and women, it is helpful to tune into this regular monthly cycle of ebb and flow as the Moon moves through the lunar cycle.

The Moon in your birth chart shows your emotional nature and how you experience life emotionally and physically. When your Moon is under stress (with challenging aspects or transits), you may feel emotionally out of balance or be vulnerable to health issues.

If your Moon has beneficial aspects, you are likely to be aware of your emotions and find it easy to express your feelings. You may be in tune with how your emotions relate to body symptoms and feel comfortable "in your own skin." You are also likely to be emotionally open and vulnerable with others as well as compassionate and caring.

If your Moon has challenging aspects, you may find it more difficult to understand or express your emotions. Another challenge you may experience is not being in tune with your body. You may feel disconnected from your body or ignore body symptoms that are also emotional messages about what may be stressing you in your life. With difficult natal aspects, you may also have found it difficult to feel nurtured or supported in childhood. The more challenging aspects you have, the more complicated or stressful your relationship with your mother may be. You may have a hard time nurturing yourself and others in intimate relationships. You may also feel conflicted about being a mother yourself or have issues around parenting your children.

While the Moon is reflective of your body and health in general, it is particularly associated with the fluids in your body. Just as the Moon affects the tides and waters of our planet, it influences the fluids in your body. The Moon's influence also relates to the digestive processes and how you nurture yourself physically and emotionally. In this way, its aspects and placement in your birth chart also provide information about what you experience as nurturing in your life and your early life experiences of nurturance, especially with your mother. The Moon in its association with the third eye and the pituitary gland is also connected with the endocrine system and hormones.

By understanding your moon sign and raising your vibrational level, you can live your life in an emotionally balanced way and improve your physical health. Following are some of the characteristics of the Moon in each sign; but look at Chapter Seven on the Archetypes of the Signs of the Zodiac for more in-depth information about your moon sign.

Key Phrases for the Moon in Each Sign of the Zodiac:

ARIES MOON:
Tends to be emotionally fiery, sometimes reactive, and does not hold onto grudges. May not think things through or may take action in a spontaneous way rather than tuning into emotions in a more conscious way.

TAURUS MOON:
Is emotionally grounded and nurtured by being in nature. Likes stability and may be stressed by too much change.

GEMINI MOON:
Needs to journal or dialogue with others in order to process feelings. Emotions are usually quick to change.

CANCER MOON:
Is emotionally sensitive and can be moody at times. Feelings are right near the surface. The Moon is the ruler of Cancer and is strongest in this sign.

LEO MOON:
Is generous and caring but tends to be emotionally sensitive to others' responses and can be easily hurt.

VIRGO MOON:
Tends to analyze feelings and can be self-critical. Strives towards self-improvement.

LIBRA MOON:
Values harmony and is often stressed by conflict in relationships. Tends to analyze feelings and tries to understand the feelings and needs of others.

SCORPIO MOON:
Is emotionally intense and feels things deeply, but often holds the feelings inside rather than expressing them overtly.

SAGITTARIUS MOON:
Tends to be optimistic and likes to share feelings and thoughts with others.

CAPRICORN MOON:
Is usually emotionally reserved and not always in touch with own emotions.

AQUARIUS MOON:
Tends to step back from own emotions and tries to analyze what is going on rather than getting caught up in the feelings. Often channels emotions into social concerns.

PISCES MOON:
Is dreamy, intuitive, emotionally sensitive, and easily affected by others' moods and surrounding energies.

House Placement

Locate the house of your birth chart in which your Moon

resides. The house that the Moon is in shows an area of life that is emotionally important to you. For you to be in balance emotionally, it is important to keep this as a strong area of focus in your life.

Aspects

Now locate the aspect lines that connect your Moon to other planets in your chart. Identify whether these are challenging or supportive aspects. Determine which ones feel like areas that represent difficulties for you emotionally or that signify strengths in your life. Conjunctions between the Moon and another planet may be either supportive or challenging depending on the combination and how you work with those energies. Squares and oppositions tend to be the more challenging of the aspects, while the sextiles and trines serve as the more supportive aspects.

CONJUNCTIONS

When a planet is in conjunction with the Moon, it indicates that your emotions and the energy of that planet may be merged. These conjunctions may be supportive or challenging depending on the planets involved.

MOON/MERCURY:

This is a supportive aspect and means that you are able to talk about your emotions and work them through with awareness.

MOON/VENUS:

You value relationships and are likely to be nurturing and compassionate in how you relate to others. If you are dealing with stress in a relationship, it is likely to have a profound impact on you emotionally.

MOON/MARS:

This is often a more challenging aspect and can mean being prone to anger acting out your emotions. However, if worked consciously, this can mean that your actions are in alignment with what is emotionally important to you.

MOON/JUPITER:

You are apt to be idealistic and have strong emotions and tend to be optimistic about life. It can indicate tendencies to be over-indulgent or to be disappointed due to your high expectations. You may also tend to be a giving person but sometimes over-extend yourself emotionally with others.

MOON/SATURN:

This aspect usually signifies that you did not feel emotionally understood or supported in childhood and so developed a strong persona to compensate, but you continue to deal with underlying feelings of insecurity and vulnerability.

MOON/URANUS:

You may have a tendency to be moody, unpredictable emotionally, or to "cut out" emotionally if under stress. You may also often feel as if you are different or unconventional and not easily understood by others.

MOON/NEPTUNE:

If you work this aspect consciously, it indicates a strong spiritual and intuitive nature. You are compassionate and sensitive toward others but tend to be vulnerable and may feel easily overwhelmed by your emotions. If this aspect is not worked consciously, it can also manifest as vulnerability to addictions, a tendency to get caught up in fantasies or escapism, or to be in relationships that are out of balance (for example, being in a caretaker role with others or feeling victimized by those who take advantage of your sensitive and giving nature).

MOON/PLUTO:
You are likely to have an intense emotional nature and a vulnerability to depression or ways of sabotaging yourself emotionally. You are likely to read emotions easily and to sense what is going on beneath the surface in interactions with others. When worked consciously, this gives you inner strength and the capacity to work through intense emotional experiences, knowing that these experiences lead to transformation and a deepening understanding of yourself.

Challenging Aspects to the Moon

SQUARES
When a planet is squaring the Moon, it is in conflict with the energy of the Moon and may indicate an emotional or health challenge. The key to emotional and physical balance is to integrate this aspect of yourself in a conscious way.

MOON/MERCURY:
You may experience a conflict between your heart and your head or between your emotions and your thoughts. If integrated, this is a strong combination and supports you in effectively communicating your feelings and being aware of your emotions.

MOON/VENUS:
You are likely to experience a tension between what you feel and need emotionally and how you behave in relationships. The challenge is to work consciously with your emotions and to choose relationships with discernment.

MOON/MARS:

You may have a tendency to be somewhat reactive, quick to anger, or overly sensitive to conflict. It will be important to learn how to work with your energy and anger in a constructive and conscious way.

MOON/JUPITER:

You are apt to be idealistic, have high expectations, and may be easily disappointed. This means that you have a strong faith and intrinsic optimism but may over-extend or over-indulge yourself at times.

MOON/SATURN:

This aspect generally means that you grew up not feeling emotionally supported or understood. You may have experienced conflicts with your mother in particular. You may be self-critical and need to learn how to honor your underlying feelings and vulnerabilities and be compassionate with yourself.

MOON/URANUS:

You may be moody or emotionally unpredictable with a tendency to withdraw or become reactive when stressed. You may also experience a conflict between your longing for independence and your need for security or connection with others.

MOON/NEPTUNE:

You are most likely sensitive, compassionate, and intuitive, but may struggle with keeping healthy boundaries with others or have addiction issues.

MOON/PLUTO:

You are likely to be intense and vulnerable to depression. You may have experienced your mother as aggressive and may get caught in power struggles with others. It is important to honor your intensity and your own issues around power and powerlessness.

OPPOSITIONS

When a planet is opposite the Moon, you may tend to disown this part of yourself and see it in others or experience it through a relationship. The challenge is to integrate this as an aspect of yourself. Oppositions with the outermost planets are the most challenging.

MOON/MERCURY:

If polarized, you may have difficulty expressing your emotions or you may seek out others to mirror your feelings and help you to understand them. If integrated, this allows you to express your emotions effectively through dialogue with others, or in your own inner process, or through writing.

MOON/VENUS:

You may experience some tension between your emotional needs and your relationships. It will be important to allow yourself to acknowledge your feelings and needs and balance that with your care and concern for those you love.

MOON/MARS:

This aspect indicates both a need to act on what you feel and a tendency to get into conflicts with others. You may have difficulties acknowledging your own feelings of anger and may tend to see this emotion in others but not as easily in yourself.

MOON/JUPITER:

You may seek to find others (teachers, mentors, guides) who encourage or inspire you, yet you need to integrate your own faith and understanding of life and your own beliefs.

MOON/SATURN:

You may experience others as controlling or critical. It is important to take in your own inner authority and find your own center.

MOON/URANUS:

You may be drawn to others who are creative and unconventional, and you may need to acknowledge those aspects of yourself.

MOON/NEPTUNE:

You are likely to be highly sensitive, empathic, and easily influenced by the feelings of others. It is important to be clear with your emotional boundaries and be careful about getting into relationships in which you become the emotional caretaker but neglect your own feelings and needs.

MOON/PLUTO:

This aspect indicates a tendency to be involved in intense relationships or experiences and to struggle with how stressful this is for you. It is important for you to acknowledge your own depth and emotional intensity without seeking out dramatic or intense interactions with others to find these aspects of yourself.

Supportive Aspects to the Moon

SEXTILES AND TRINES

Conjunctions with the Moon may be either challenging or supportive depending on the energy of the planet and how you integrate this facet of yourself, the sextiles and trines are the most supportive aspects and indicate emotional strengths. The sextiles are generally gifts or strengths that you are conscious of in yourself, while the trines indicate more intrinsic (and less conscious) aspects of who you are. Following are some of the ways that these supportive aspects of the Moon and a planet may manifest in your life.

MOON/MERCURY:

You are likely to be comfortable in communicating your feelings verbally or in writing. Dialoguing with another person or journal writing is a good avenue for getting in touch with or processing your emotions.

MOON/VENUS:

This usually indicates that you value relationships and are emotionally open with others. Your emotions are easily influenced by what is going on in your relationships.

MOON/MARS:

This shows that you are likely to be assertive and comfortable with expressing your anger effectively with others. You also may use exercise to release emotional or physical stress. Your actions are an expression of your emotions and demonstrate what you care about in your life.

MOON/JUPITER:

You tend to be optimistic and may have a strong sense of faith that things will work out in a positive manner even when they seem challenging in the moment. You tend to be generous and giving with others.

MOON/SATURN:

This indicates a strong inner self and an ability to have good boundaries emotionally. You are likely to be steady and grounded emotionally and not easily overwhelmed by stress or emotions.

MOON/URANUS:

You value truth and authenticity, are honest with your emotions, and you value that in others. You are apt to be perceptive and value getting to the heart of what is going on in yourself and others emotionally.

MOON/NEPTUNE:
This indicates a compassionate, empathic, and caring nature and strong intuition. You may be tuned into your dreams and understand how they are an effective way of processing your emotions. You are emotionally sensitive and easily influenced by music, and you have a strong mystical aspect to who you are.

MOON/PLUTO:
You are likely to feel things in a deep and intense manner and value deep relationships. You are able to sense what others are feeling even if they are not expressing their feelings in a direct or open manner. Others may feel safe in sharing their secrets or deep feelings and experiences with you.

Examples of Moon Signs and Their Aspects

In order to see how these aspects manifest, we will explore the primary aspects to the Moon in Allie's chart as well as in the charts of Oprah Winfrey and Deepak Chopra.

Moon Sign and House Placement: According to her birth chart, Allie's moon sign is in Cancer like her sun sign. The Moon is strongest in this sign, and this supports Allie in being emotionally aware and in tune with her body. It also strengthens her sun sign's qualities of being emotionally sensitive and caring. Her Moon is in the tenth house, which means that her career is important to her emotionally, and she needs to be in a job that she can truly put her heart into. If her work is not a good fit for her, this will be very stressful for her emotionally and physically.

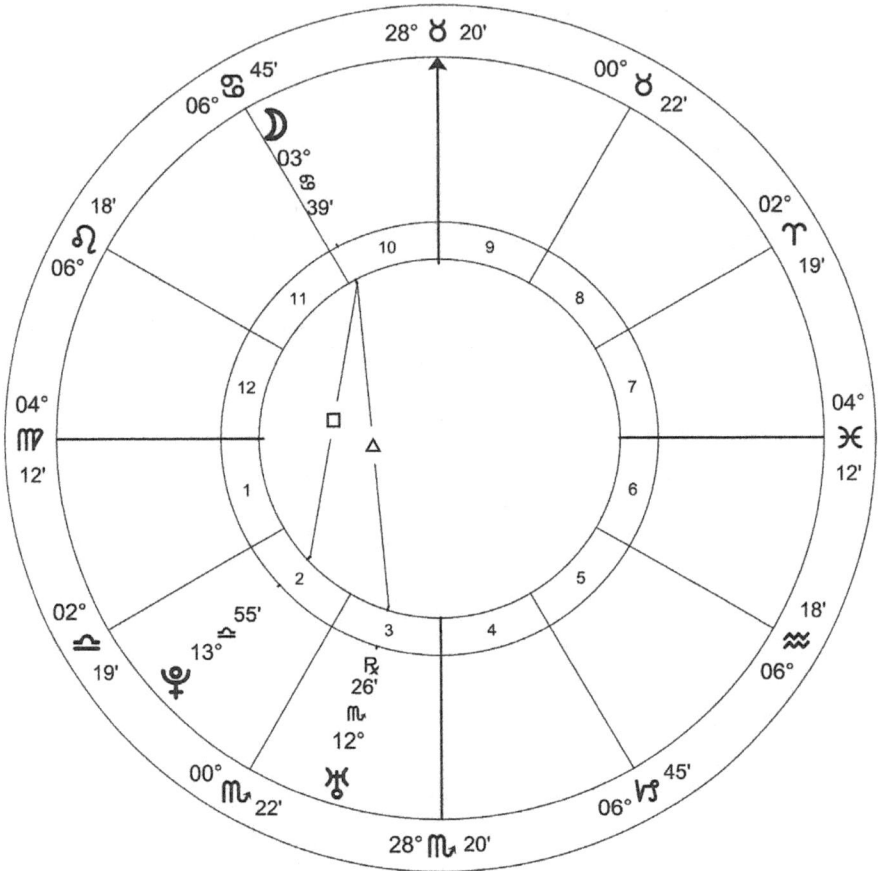

Allie's Chart with Moon Aspects

Aspects to the Moon: Like her Sun, Allie's Moon in her birth chart is in strong aspects to both Pluto and Uranus. The challenging aspect (a square) to Pluto indicates that she feels things very deeply. She may have a tendency to keep trying to work things through even when it is not good for her emotionally. By being self-aware and finding a way to keep this aspect in balance, she can honor her intensity and put her energies into situations that are healthy for her rather than staying too long in stressful situations that negatively impact her emotions and health. The aspect of the Moon with Uranus (trine) can guide Allie to listen to her emotions and to realize that stress and frustration are emotional signals that she may be in situations that are not a good fit for her and that are not healthy.

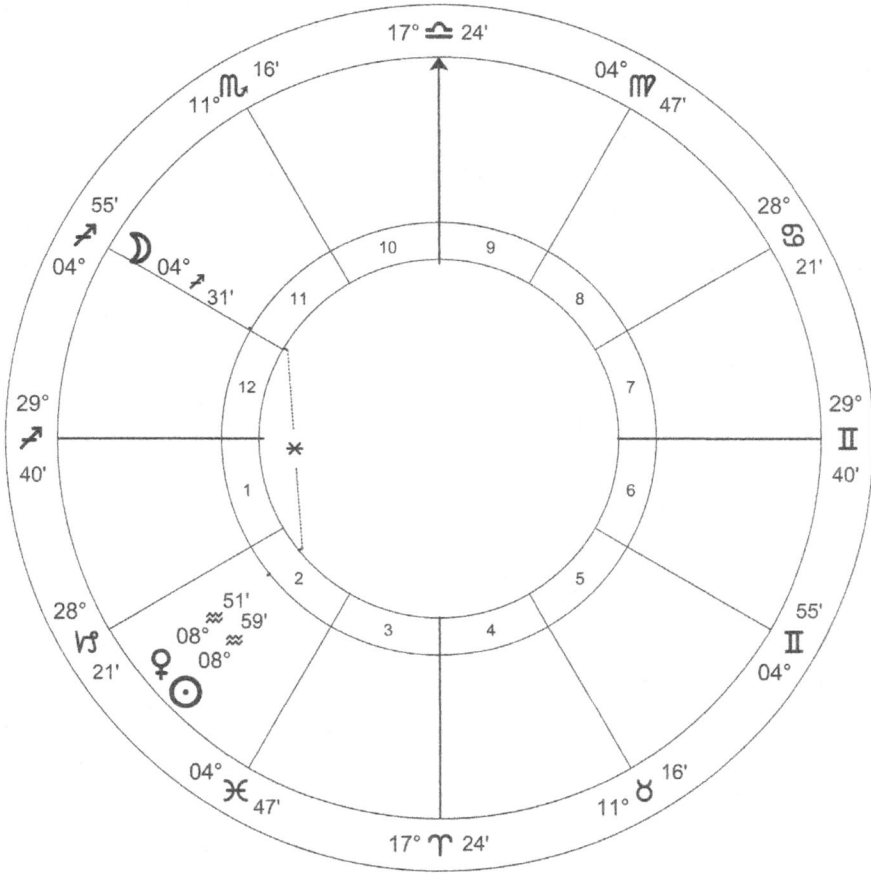

Oprah Winfrey's Chart with Moon Aspects

Oprah's Moon Sign and House Placement: In her birth chart, Oprah's Moon is in Sagittarius, indicating a love of learning, gifts in communication and teaching, and a concern with understanding life from a philosophical or spiritual perspective. The placement of her Moon in the 11th house reflects a strong interest in groups, in social issues, and in achieving her goals. It also suggests that she is extroverted in nature and that her friendships are emotionally important to her. The Moon is right on the cusp between the 11th and 12th houses. With its connection to the 12th house, this can indicate a feeling that her mother was in some ways not fully present or available to her (as was the case in her early history). It also indicates a strong imagination and sensitive nature.

Aspects to the Moon: The Moon is in a supportive aspect (sextile) to Venus in Oprah's chart, which highlights how much she values friendships and relationships. Being emotionally engaged with others is important to her in her life and in her work.

In Chinese medicine, the Moon in Sagittarius relates to the pericardium organ, which corresponds with how digestion influences hormones and energy production. The sextile from the natal Sun and Venus conjunction further supports the influences discussed earlier from the Jupiter aspect with her Sun and Venus. This Moon placement makes Oprah prone to emotional eating. How she feels at the time she eats will affect how she digests her food. This continued theme of supporting healthy digestion and emotional eating patterns is always present for Oprah in her life.

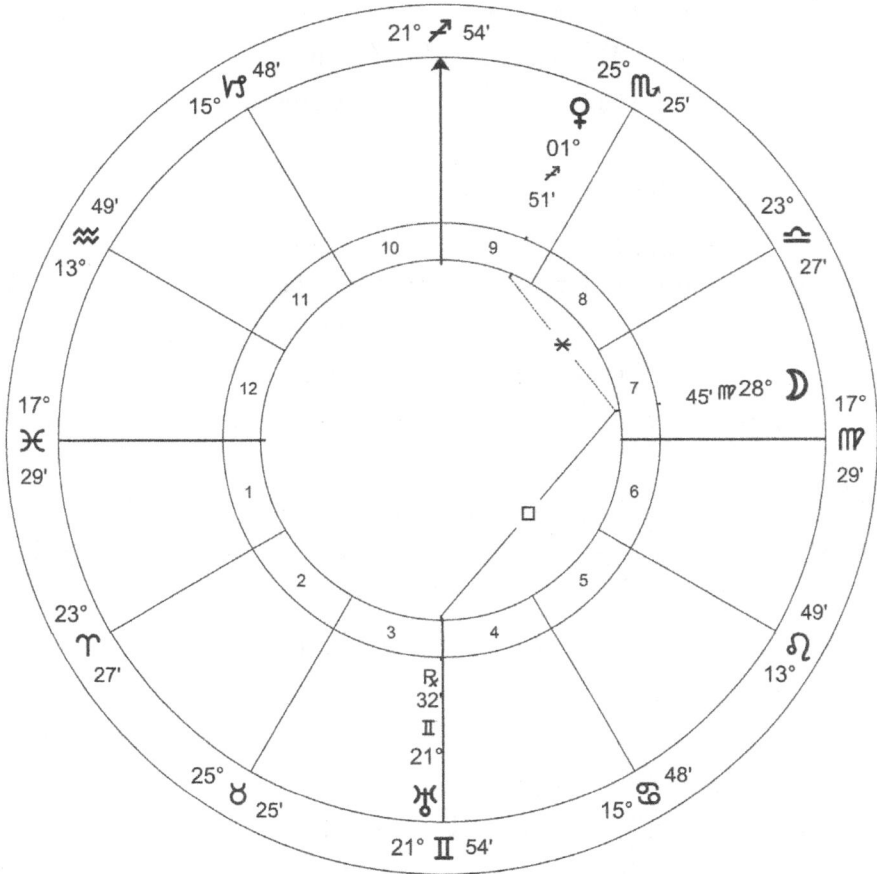

Deepak Chopra's Chart with Moon Aspects

Deepak's Moon Sign and House Placement: Deepak's Moon is in Virgo in his birth chart, indicating that he has a strong interest in health from an integrative perspective and desires to be of service to others. Being in the seventh house, his Moon shows that he values close personal relationships and that his marriage and primary relationships are crucial to his emotional well-being.

Aspects to the Moon: Like Oprah, Deepak's Moon is in a supportive aspect to Venus indicating that he also values relationships and is caring in how he engages with others. His Moon is in a more challenging aspect (square) with Uranus. This reflects that he is unconventional in his nature, values authenticity, and may also value self-awareness and attuning to his different emotions.

In Chinese medicine, the Moon in Virgo corresponds with the small intestine organ. Deepak has written several books on how mental and emotional health is directly related to digestion and our eating habits. Allopathic medicine recognizes that most neurotransmitters that control brain function are created in the small intestine. Deepak's Venus is an evening star and corresponds with the urinary bladder meridian in Chinese medicine. This is the ruler of his sun sign and further strengthens the focus of the nervous system and emotional health as a key theme in his writing.

The Uranus square to Deepak's natal Moon is in alignment with his recent books on how unhealthy emotions cause negative eating patterns and healthy recipes using whole foods and a diet high in Omega-3 fats from fish, olive oil, and avocados support people with sensitive nervous systems the best. When people eat too many other plant-based Omega-6 fats from nuts and seeds, they will likely experience increased inflammation and digestive difficulties.

The Lunar Cycle: Moon Phases and Their Meanings

Your moon sign reflects how you experience and express your emotions. The phase of the Moon that you were born into indicates how you carry the energy and theme of that time in the lunar cycle. For example, if you were born during the full Moon, you may find yourself focused on relationships and see yourself in others or find yourself mirrored by others as the full Moon mirrors the Sun. If you were born when the Moon was in conjunction with the Sun and was in its phase of invisibility just before the new Moon, you may be more introverted and reflective.

To find which phase of the Moon you were born into, look at your chart and locate the Sun. Then move around the wheel counter-clockwise until you arrive at your Moon. Count the degrees that your Moon is ahead of or behind the Sun. The Moon is ahead of the Sun if it is moving forward in the signs (but less than halfway around the wheel). The Moon is behind the Sun if between 180 and 360 degrees from the Sun.

Following are the meanings of the phases of the Moon as it moves through its monthly cycle. We tend to resonate with the phase of the lunar cycle that we were born into and carry that energy as a theme throughout our lives.

NEW MOON
(When the Moon is 0-45 degrees ahead of the Sun in the chart): this is the time in the lunar cycle for seeding new intentions or dreams and visualizing a new project or pattern. If you were born during this phase, you may be an initiator, enjoying visualizing new projects or creating new ideas, but you may not always be clear about how to bring the project into form.

CRESCENT MOON
(When the Moon is 45-90 degrees ahead of the Sun): this lunar phase is about moving forward and exploring a new project or intention. If you were born during this phase, you may enjoy the creative process, taking in new information and exploring new directions, but you may tend to move on to something new when things get challenging or be confused about what direction is right for you.

FIRST QUARTER MOON

(When the Moon is 90-135 degrees ahead of the Sun): this phase in the lunar cycle is about a crisis in action. It is about assessing how to put your intention into action and bring the project into form. If born during this phase of the Moon, you may feel pulled in different directions and have difficulty finding clarity about your path and what steps to take. You may feel some tension between your sense of your identity and your emotional nature. You feel a sense of urgency to act and to live your life with purpose but may lack confidence or be unclear about what direction to move in.

GIBBOUS MOON

(When the Moon is 135-180 degrees ahead of the Sun): this time in the lunar cycle is about analyzing and improving projects, reshaping intentions, and working out the forms or manifestation of your dreams. If you were born during this phase of the Moon, you may focus on self-improvement and on analyzing your experiences to get clearer about your direction and how you want to manifest your goals.

FULL MOON

(When the Moon is 180-135 degrees behind the Sun): this phase is about bringing projects to fullness, seeing the intention or new pattern with clarity, and experiencing the fruits of the work of the waxing half of the lunar cycle. If you were born during this phase of the Moon, you enjoy bringing projects to completion. You also enjoy being in relationships with others and mirroring them or being seen by them, much as the Moon mirrors the Sun at the time of the full Moon.

DISSEMINATING MOON

(When the Moon is 135-90 degrees behind the Sun): this is the time for sharing the project or new insights with others and letting this new project or pattern be of service in the world. If you were born during this phase, you may feel a strong desire to bring your gifts out in a visible way and to make an impact in the world.

LAST QUARTER MOON

(When the Moon is 90-45 degrees behind the Sun): this lunar phase is about a crisis in consciousness. You have now completed the project or pattern, and this is a time for reorienting, letting go, and moving on from your attachment or identification with this intention or project. If you were born during this phase of the Moon, you may struggle with your beliefs and what you identify with, feeling the limitations of any model or form.

BALSAMIC MOON

(When the Moon is 45-0 degrees behind the Sun): this is the time for integrating the lessons learned from this lunar cycle, and the time for releasing the projects or intentions that you have completed. If you were born during this phase, you tend to be reflective, integrating your experiences and seeing the bigger picture without attaching to the outcome. You realize that life is a cycle and that everything is in a process of life/death/rebirth.

Chart example: Allie's Moon is close to her Sun and is in the balsamic phase. This shows her ability to reflect on her life and to see things in a larger context. She understands that everything is in a cycle of change but may struggle to know how to move into the changes that she seeks for herself personally and professionally.

The Natal Moon Sign and the Conception Vessel

In Chinese medicine, the Moon relates to hormonal balance and the endocrine system; its importance cannot be overstated. Hormones interact with every other system in the body, strongly influence emotional health, and are critical for men and women of all ages. Natal aspects to the Moon, along with the current planetary transits, influence transition from adolescence to childbearing years and again into menopause and andropause (male menopause). The lunar cycle strongly influences women during their reproductive years because of the special relationship between the monthly menstrual cycle and the phases of the Moon.

As seen with the natal Sun, the natal Moon relates to the conception vessel that forms when the sperm enters the egg, and the first cells divide. The conception vessel is yin, feminine, and controls the yin meridians of the body. The conception vessel relates to blood and the essence needed to give form to a new being. In Chinese medicine, the mother's role in creating new life holds greater importance than the man's contribution because the mother's soul *Po* allows the child's spirit to enter the Earth through the breath. Therefore, the mother's ability to oxygenate the blood allows the soul of the unborn baby to integrate with the baby's body before birth.

In Chinese medicine, the conception vessel, known as the "Sea of Yin Channels," includes the reproductive organs for both men and women and controls puberty; it initiates the seeds of life and the creative drive. The conception vessel directs the pituitary to create sperm in men and to mature follicles and eggs in women. Yin strongly influences women; thus, this vessel initiates the menstrual cycle and later in life the transition into menopause.

The conception vessel rules the pituitary gland and pairs with the governing vessel, which relates to the hypothalamus gland. The hypothalamus-pituitary axis creates the foundation for the entire endocrine system, which corresponds with these paired vessels. The hypothalamus and governing vessel direct the pituitary and the conception vessel to run the endocrine system. The Moon reflects the light of the Sun and, in turn, expresses emotions. Harmonizing the Sun and Moon influences our physical and emotional health and is most important for the healthy expression of our identity.

The source of creativity and the seeds of reproduction are both associated with the conception vessel. The expression "birthing a project" refers to the creative process that brings life to our heart's desires. Whether you are supporting your Moon for emotional health, focusing on the Moon's ruling of the reproductive system, or expressing your creativity in other areas, try incorporating the Natal Moon Luminary Blend with the other planetary or sign blends.

The Natal Moon Luminary Blend supports coming into balance with the planetary aspects in your chart. By combining the Natal Moon Luminary Blend with a challenging planetary aspect blend, you can positively integrate uncomfortable situations and emotions instead of feeling blocked or constricted. If your Sun and Moon are in a challenging aspect to each other, then combining the Natal Moon Luminary Blend with your sun sign blend can help harmonize your feelings with your sense of identity. By combining the Natal Moon Luminary Blend with another beneficial planetary aspect blend, you can enhance your creativity and harness the positive energies of the associated aspect.

In her birth chart, Allie's natal Moon is in the sign of Cancer with a square (challenging aspect) to the planet Pluto and a trine (beneficial aspect) to the planet Uranus. When Allie feels frustrated or is unable to express her emotions in positive ways, she can combine the Natal Moon Luminary Blend with the Pluto Planetary Blend to help her consciously work through challenging feelings. When Allie is working on creative projects and expressing herself in new ways, she can combine the Natal Moon Luminary Blend with the Uranus Planetary Blend to enhance her clarity and creativity.

The Harmonizing Essence of the Natal Moon Luminary Blend

The Natal Moon Luminary Blend (also known as the Ren/ Conception Vessel Meridian Balancing Blend) consists of 50% lavender (*Lavandula angustifolia*), 25% black pepper (*Piper nigrum*), and 25% myrrh (*Commiphora myrrha*). This blend combines well with other oils and blends. In addition to reflecting the light of the Sun, the Moon also tends to mirror energy from the planets that are in aspect with it. The Natal Moon Luminary Blend works best when combined with a planetary blend in aspect to the Moon. Try smelling this blend with other oils or other important blends based on your chart, and your intuition will guide you to the right mix.

Lavender essential oil harmonizes with other oils, adapts to the immediate needs of the body, and cleanses the hormone receptor sites that are commonly congested with xenoestrogens found in plastics from our environment. Lavender's versatility makes it the perfect oil to support emotional health by calming the nervous system and encouraging us to adapt to life's challenges. Lavender optimizes estrogen, the dominant hormone in women, by cleansing the receptor sites that are clogged with environmental toxins in the form of xenoestrogens and supporting healthy levels. In men, it is important that estrogen balances their dominant hormone, testosterone, for both emotional health and physical endurance. Today, everyone is constantly exposed to xenoestrogens in our environment that disrupt neurotransmitters, hormones, and emotional health. In the Natal Moon Luminary Blend, lavender helps to cleanse and soothe emotional wounds while harmonizing the other oils combined with it.

Folklore tells us that for thousands of years before the birth of Jesus Christ, myrrh was one of the most expensive and desired oils in the world. Myrrh has strong ties to Christianity, and the three wise men (also astrologers) presented it to Jesus at his birth. Myrrh was again offered to Christ to relieve his pain while he was dying on the cross, and large amounts of myrrh anointed his body at his burial. Catholic Masses and gatherings regularly burn myrrh and frankincense resin in honor of the birth of Jesus Christ. In Chinese medicine today, myrrh resin, known as *mo yao*, regulates blood flow, reduces swelling, alleviates, pain, and promotes healing. *Mo yao* affects the heart, liver, and spleen meridians, which correspond with the transiting Sun and Moon, and the planet Neptune.

Myrrh essential oil is a thick resin and is best used in small amounts as it amplifies the effects of other oils mixed with it. Myrrh essential oil supports healthy hormone levels and reproductive organs, beautifies the skin, and supports emotional balance. Black pepper, surprisingly, balances myrrh's intense aroma.

Black pepper essential oil supplies oxygen to the cells and stimulates the brain, which balances the calming effects of lavender and myrrh. Black pepper oil connects the mind and the reproductive organs to promote healthy sexual and creative expression. This oil is commonly added to both aphrodisiac blends and blends that enhance creativity. Myrrh also, surprisingly, balances black pepper's intense aroma.

How to Use the Natal Moon Luminary Blend

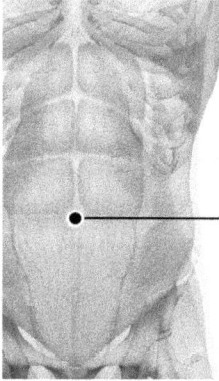

CV-8
Spirit
Gateway
(Umbilicus)

There are two important acupuncture points along the conception vessel: Spirit Gateway and Origin Pass. Spirit Gateway, also known as *Shen Que*, Spirit Palace, Conception Vessel 8, or CV-8, is found directly in the middle of the umbilicus (the belly button). Chinese medicine believes this acupuncture point is where the spirit both enters and exits the body. Needling Spirit Gateway in acupuncture is forbidden, but heating it with a special herb called moxa, commonly known as mugwort or *ai ye* is acceptable. Additionally, Spirit Gateway naturally forms a reservoir that perfectly holds essential oils. In Michelle Meramour's Body-Feedback style of acupuncture, this point is recognized as being constantly sensitive or tender to the touch when the soul or the body experienced trauma in the womb or during the birthing process. It can also become tender during times of extreme physical and emotional stress. When tender, Spirit Gateway reveals that the body is in fight or flight mode. Applying the correct essential oil blend on the point is the most effective way to release the prenatal or birth trauma as well as the current stressors affecting emotional health.

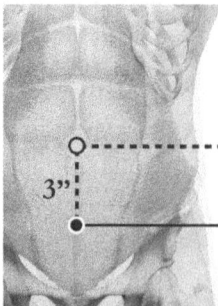

3"

Umbilicus

CV-4
Origin Pass

Origin Pass, also known as *Guan Yuan*, Conception Vessel 4, or CV-4, is found three inches below the umbilicus, or Spirit Gateway, at the same level as the corresponding Life Gate point found on the governing vessel. Origin Pass refers to the "passageway of original *qi*" or the place where "original *qi* is stored [locked in]." [1] This point corresponds to the level of the second chakra and the uterus for women. Applying the Natal Moon Luminary Blend to Origin Pass can help give form to creative ideas and support a healthy expression of sexuality. Accessing this point also supports reflecting on emotions and the world around us.

Note: Always dilute the essential oils applied in the belly button due to possible skin sensitivities to the oils. If you are experiencing stress or have a strained relationship with your mother or children, applying essential oils to Spirit Gateway may bring you surprising relief and self-reflection to process these emotions in a beneficial way.

Natal Moon Luminary Affirmations:	I am in tune with what I feel. I nurture myself and am caring with others. I am in tune with the rhythms of nature and of my body

---

[1] Andrew Ellis, Nigel Wiseman, and Ken Boss, *Grasping the Wind* (Brookline: Paradigm Publications, 1989), 307.

The Transiting Sun and Moon

The core themes and planetary aspects in your birth chart are with you throughout your lifetime. How you work with these energy patterns, and how they manifest in your life can change significantly as you deepen your self-awareness, progress in inner healing, and increase your vibrational level. While the birth chart stays the same throughout your life, you are influenced by the energies of the Sun, Moon, and planets as they move in the sky and circle around your birth chart activating different points or aspects in your chart. The movements of the planets and their interactions with your chart are called "transits." As different transiting planets activate parts of your chart, these transits bring those energies or planetary aspects in your natal chart into your awareness. They give you the opportunity to heal or transform those areas of your life. While we will not go into depth with all of the planetary transits in this book, we will help you to understand and work with the energies of the transiting Sun and Moon.

The Sun and Moon, as they move through their dance together in the sky, carry us through the energies of each lunar cycle as well as the seasonal cycle. As these luminaries travel around our natal charts, they bring their energy and light to different aspects in our charts, affecting each of us in a unique way.

You can find where the transiting Sun and Moon are influencing your life and your birth chart by checking on the current positions of the Sun and Moon, either through an online astrology website or through an astrologer. Note where the Sun and Moon line up with that same sign and degree in your chart. You now are able to see the houses that are being activated by these luminaries as well as any planets or aspects that they are illuminating.

Remember that the Sun moves one degree around the wheel each day so that it will be in each sign and house for about thirty days. The Moon moves more rapidly and travels thirteen degrees per day so that it will be in each sign and house for a little less than three days. The movement of the Sun guides us through the annual seasonal cycle, while the dance of the Moon in relationship with the Sun carries us through the lunar or monthly cycle.

The Transiting Sun and the Heart Meridian

As the Sun moves through the seasonal cycle, it affects our energy levels and moods as we feel the shifting of temperature and of light and dark. You might experience seasonal affective disorder, with increased feelings of depression and exhaustion as the sunlight decreases in the late fall and winter. It is also common to feel an increase in energy and uplifting of mood as the sunlight returns after the spring equinox and continues to increase through the summer months. Using the Transiting Sun Luminary Blend can help you adapt to the shifting seasonal energies and the changes in light and dark.

As the Sun moves through the different signs and houses, it will highlight various parts of your chart and facets of who you are. These are times when the light of awareness can help you to see those parts of yourself more fully. The transits of the Sun may highlight areas of stress or unresolved issues in your life. Using the Transiting Sun Luminary Blend can help you open up to and more effectively integrate the energies of that sign and of the planets in your chart that are being illuminated.

The Earth's rotation around the Sun marks both the diurnal cycle as well as the seasonal cycle. It teaches us each day about the dance of light and dark and of new beginnings and endings with the energy of the sunrise and sunset. Each evening, we experience the death of the Sun and see its rebirth at sunrise. In this way, working with the transiting Sun also helps us to move through times of transition in our lives and to remember that the light returns after even the longest and darkest nights when we feel overwhelmed, depressed, or stressed.

In Chinese medicine, the heart organ stores the soul while sleeping, and the transiting Sun can influence your quality of sleep. The hypothalamus and pituitary glands work together to generate the proper balance of cortisol and melatonin, which regulate the energy cycle in the body and are dependent on daylight and darkness. The seasonal cycle strongly influences the sleep cycle based on the length of sunlight during the day. The Transiting Sun Luminary Blend harmonizes and supports a healthy hypothalamus and pituitary connection, influencing the sleep cycle and emotional health.

If you have a fire sun sign such as Aries, Leo, or Sagittarius, you may find that you sleep better in the winter when there is less light or by making time to exercise during the day if you do not have an active job. If you have an earth sun sign, such as Taurus, Virgo, or Capricorn, you may find a light snack before bed, or a relaxing walk outside encourages a good night sleep. If you have an air sun sign, such as Gemini, Libra, or Aquarius, you might find reading a book or watching a little television in the evening is a gentle way to stimulate the mind before bed during the shorter days and may need yoga to clear your mind in summer when the days are long. If you have a water sun sign, such as Cancer, Scorpio, or Pisces, you might enjoy an evening bath with mineral salts or ocean sounds to meditate with before bed.

The Harmonizing Essence of the Transiting Sun Luminary Blend

The Transiting Sun Luminary Blend (also known as the Heart Meridian Balancing Blend) consists of 50% ylang ylang (*Cananga odorata*), 25% sacred frankincense (*Boswellia sacra*), and 25% frankincense (*Boswellia carterii*). The family of frankincense oils comes from the resin of the tree bark. The higher quality oils are clear to silvery in color, and the lower quality oils are darker brown in color. The synergy of the standard frankincense along with sacred frankincense supports a balanced endocrine system by strengthening the hypothalamus and pituitary connection. These master glands of the endocrine system strongly influence emotional health, including how we process and handle daily stressors and life-changing events.

The different species of frankincense affect the meridian system differently. The standard frankincense supports more of the yang, masculine, energizing, and warming functions in the body. The sacred frankincense supports more of the yin, feminine, calming, and harmonizing function in the body. When blending different species of the same plant family together, they almost always need another harmonizing oil to bring together their healing properties. In this blend, ylang ylang harmonizes the different frankincense species and allows the blend to adapt to your needs in the moment.

Ylang ylang, a tropical evergreen, can grow to a height of 100 feet and blooms almost year round. The mature ylang ylang tree resembles a traditional Christmas tree or northern hemisphere evergreen. Ylang ylang and the family of frankincense oils are the strongest of the adaptogenic oils, which can help us adapt to challenging situations we find ourselves in thereby allowing us to approach life with stable emotions and a poised heart chakra. All three of these oils are highly beneficial for the skin and have strong anti-aging properties to help keep you young at heart.

How to Use the Transiting Sun Luminary Blend

Applying the diluted blend directly over the heart area supports emotional health and the endocrine system during stressful times. Diluting this blend with a facial carrier oil creates a beautiful facial serum for a youthful complexion and can help you adjust to both daily transitions and life-changing events. Diffusing this blend can help you adjust to difficult times and major life transitions including birth and death. Because of the adaptogenic nature of this blend, homemade skin care and shower gels using this blend make perfect holiday gifts.

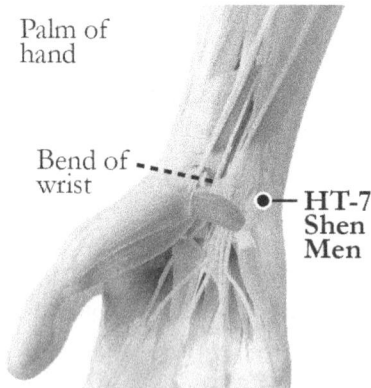

Palm of hand

Bend of wrist

●—HT-7
Shen
Men

The most common acupuncture point used to support emotional health during challenging times is *Shen Men*, commonly known as Spirit Gate or Heart 7. This point is found on the palmar side of the wrist crease at the head of the ulnar bone and just inside the ulnar tendon. This famous acupuncture point addresses emotional stress affecting the spirit and adds energy to the meridian to strengthen the spirit because it is a special source point. This point treats disorders of the spirit including mania, poor memory, and insomnia, and is a "gateway" to treating the spirit. Spirit Gate is an earth point on the fire meridian that helps to control and balance the fire element. It helps ground your spirit and to feel at home on the Earth plane. Applying the Transiting Sun Luminary Blend, also known as the Heart Meridian Balancing Blend, directly to Spirit Gate can help you adjust to stressful times and replenish your spirit energy as you travel along your soul's journey here on Earth.

Affirmations for the Transiting Sun Luminary Blend:	I open my heart to gratitude for the present moment. I see myself clearly and feel centered even in the midst of change. I open to the healing heat and light of the Sun to fill me with energy and uplift my spirit.

The Transiting Moon and the Spleen Meridian

The Moon moves through the sky more rapidly than the Sun and any of the other planets since it circles close to our Earth. Since it moves thirteen degrees in our charts each day, it is in one sign and one house for a little less than three days before moving to the next sign and house. We feel both its shifting energy with the sign that it is in as well as the shifting rhythms of the lunar cycle and how that affects our bodies and moods. The pull of the Moon on the Earth and the tides and its influence on our moods and hormones are greatest at the time of the new Moon and full Moon. It is well known that we may be more introspective or reflective at the time of the new Moon and are likely to feel more flooded with emotions at the time of the full Moon. For women during their reproductive years who are in tune with the lunar cycle, menstruation occurs at the time of the new Moon and ovulation at the time of the full Moon.

For all of us, the new Moon is a time to set intentions for the coming month, which we can then act on through the time of the waxing Moon. We will experience these intentions coming to fruition at the time of the full Moon. As the Moon wanes in her cycle, we share what we have learned or the fruits of our intentions with others, reflect on this experience, and allow ourselves to let go of this focus as the Moon completes its cycle.

As the Moon moves through the signs, it touches different planets in your chart and may bring up unresolved emotions or activate bodily sensations. You may feel more enlivened when the Moon is in a fire sign and more emotional when it moves through a water sign. You may feel a need to talk about your emotions when it is in an air sign or feel more grounded and in touch with your body when it is in an earth sign. Also, note which house the Moon is in as it moves around your chart. The house placement shows the area of life in which you will feel the energy of the Moon activating emotions or issues for you.

In Chinese medicine, the spleen meridian relates to the transiting Moon, the pancreas, and the spleen organ. The Chinese function of the spleen includes carbohydrate and sugar digestion, blood sugar regulation, energy production, and immune system functions. The spleen meridian changes its role throughout the day to meet your immediate needs. Stress, irregular eating, consuming too much sugar, and over-exercising can all disrupt the spleen meridian and encourage moodiness.

The Harmonizing Essence of the Transiting Moon Luminary Blend

The Transiting Moon Luminary Blend (also known as the Spleen Meridian Balancing Blend) consists of 50% orange (*Citrus sinensis*), 25% clove (*Syzygium aromaticum*), and 25% copaiba (copal: *Copaifera reticulate* or *Copaifera L. genus*). The synergistic effect of these three oils supports digestion, regulates blood sugar, and lessens the negative physical and emotional effects of sugar. Orange essential oil supports the lymph system, aids in the first stages of digestion, and regulates the fluids in the body. In Chinese medicine, medicinal herbs made from oranges respond in the same way as the essential oil and control dampness, which comes from stagnant fluids and a diet too high in carbohydrates.

Clove essential oil cleanses the cellular receptor sites, protects the body by supporting a healthy immune system response, and aids the body in completing the normal and healthy inflammatory response needed for regeneration. Clove essential oil is beneficial for any symptom made worse with diets high in sugar and carbohydrates. Clove oil is high in phenols, which can irritate sensitive skin, but is helpful when taken internally.

Copaiba essential oil enhances the effects of the clove and orange oils while providing digestive support. Copaiba has a slightly sweet aroma and also supports stable blood sugar and a healthy inflammatory cycle. In addition, copaiba is high in sesquiterpenes to support brain function and emotional health. Copaiba combined with orange and clove in this blend will help stabilize your mood and offers stable energy when you have to skip meals or wait too long to eat.

How to Use the Transiting Moon Luminary Blend

The Transiting Moon Luminary Blend can support the early stages of digestion and help stabilize blood sugar if you find yourself waiting too long between meals. This blend benefits the digestive system and is best taken with meals internally if the manufacturer and FDA approve your oils for internal use. Adding a few drops to a glass of water, or to a capsule, can aid your digestion and enzyme production while keeping your energy stable.

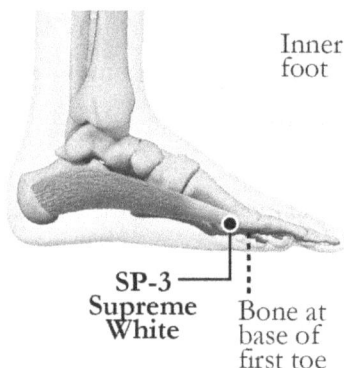

Inner foot

SP-3
Supreme White

Bone at base of first toe

The acupuncture point Supreme White, also known as *Tai Bai*, Spleen 3, or SP-3, references the Chinese name for the planet of Venus. As a morning star, Venus relates to the sweetness of life and specifically to sugar and carbohydrate consumption. Supreme White is found along the inside border of the foot's arch, just behind the largest bone at the base of the first toe where the color and texture of the skin changes dramatically. Acupuncturists use Supreme White to reduce sugar cravings and harmonize the spleen meridian.

Applying the Transiting Moon Luminary Blend to the soles of the feet, with a focus on the acupuncture point Supreme White, is preferred for this blend because it includes a citrus oil that can increase photosensitivity and clove that can irritate the skin. Starting the day by supporting energy production and blood sugar regulation with this blend on Supreme White will help you find the sweetness in your daily activities and lessen the need for sugary foods.

Affirmations for the Transiting Moon Luminary Blend:

I go with the flow and stay fluid in how I deal with life.

I listen to my own rhythms and am in tune with the cycles of the Moon.

I honor my changing emotions and listen to the messages from my body.

Guide to Higher Vibrational Living

*I've worked all my life on the subject of awareness,
whether it's awareness of the body, awareness of the mind,
awareness of your emotions, awareness of your relationships,
or awareness of your environment. I think the key to transforming
your life is to be aware of who you are.*

—Deepak Chopra

Now that you have become familiar with your Sun and Moon and the signs they are in, as well as their important planetary aspects, you can use the steps below to support being more in balance physically and emotionally. As you align with your true self and consciously integrate the energies of your Sun and Moon, you will raise your vibrational level energetically.

For each of the steps below, we recommend taking one month to work with the appropriate oils. This allows time to integrate the changes brought about by nourishing your spirit through astrology, essential oils, and Chinese medicine.

Some blends work better together than others, based on the individual ingredients. As you begin working with your natal chart and the associated blends, take a moment to smell a blend separately, then with other blends to make sure their combined aroma is appealing to you. You will have a natural attraction to the individual and combined blends when they are beneficial to you and are harmonizing your Sun and Moon in your natal chart.

Below are some suggested protocols that will help you increase your energy vibration through the integration of the oil blends with your Sun and Moon signs:

Basic Protocol

1.   Use the sign oil blend that your Sun is in to support you in your sense of self, your confidence in your gifts, and your ability to live out who you are to the fullest. Use this oil blend on any of the points described in this book that relate to the Sun or your Sun sign, or apply the oil to your heart or third eye. Use the affirmations associated with this sign to help you more fully align with your true self and the way in which you bring your light into the world. Try doing this daily for one month.

2.   Use the sign oil blend that your Moon is in to heal and to support you emotionally. Use this oil blend on any of the points for the Moon or your Moon sign, or apply the oil to your heart. Use the affirmations associated with this sign to allow yourself to hold yourself in love and compassion and to honor all that

you feel and who you are in this life. Apply the oil blend and use the affirmations daily for a month, ideally beginning with a New Moon and continuing through one full lunar cycle.

3.   If there is a challenging aspect in your chart to either your Sun or your Moon, take a month and use the planetary blend for the challenging planet daily to connect with that energy and to more fully integrate the gifts of this planet rather than feeling blocked or in conflict with it. Use the affirmations related to this planet or the sign that it is in to more fully connect with and integrate that energy as part of who you are.

4.   If you are dealing with a particular issue in your life, find the planet or sign that resonates with that issue, then use that planetary or sign blend and the associated affirmations for a month to support you in working with that issue. For example, if you are struggling with speaking your truth, use the Mercury planetary blend to support your self-expression. If you need to feel more grounded in your life, use the Taurus sign blend to help you to feel more stable, secure and centered. If you feel that you lack energy, use the Mars planetary blend or Aries sign blend to energize you.

Advanced Protocol

If you would like to work in greater depth with the challenging and supportive aspects to your natal Sun and Moon, use this protocol to raise your vibrational level and harmonize the energies of your Sun and Moon. This protocol guides you in more fully clearing blocks and inner conflicts as well as in integrating your strengths and gifts.

Note that it may be valuable to journal about your experience while working with each of the steps below. This time of reflection can help solidify the changes you are making in your life. By highlighting the emotions and changes you experience, you will know the most appropriate blends to work with later on, if you find yourself again dealing with similar challenges or processing similar emotions.

1. WORKING WITH THE SUN AND MOON
   SIGN BLENDS

First, use the basic protocol described above to honor and integrate the energies of your Sun and Moon signs. This supports you in being true to the essence of who you are and your emotional nature, and lays the foundation for working more deeply with the challenging and supportive aspects in your chart.

Next, work on the challenging aspects in your chart, to clear the blocks and inner conflicts expressed in these aspects. Then you can integrate the supportive aspects to more fully integrate your gifts and inner strengths.

2. WORKING WITH THE CHALLENGING ASPECTS TO YOUR SUN OR MOON

Working with the challenging aspects to your Sun and Moon from your chart will harmonize these energies or frequencies and help you to fully integrate the gifts of each planet rather than feeling blocked or in conflict with it. Using affirmations will help you assimilate the wisdom acquired by working through the challenging aspects and strengthen your expression of your Sun and Moon signs. Use the essential oils on whichever acupuncture points relate to the planet, your natal Sun or Moon, or your Sun or Moon sign. Alternatively, you can apply the oils to the soles of your feet or spine.

In general, a planet squaring the Sun or Moon is likely to be the most challenging aspect to the luminaries. Oppositions or conjunctions with the outermost planets (Uranus, Neptune, and Pluto) or with Chiron are typically the next most challenging, followed by oppositions or conjunctions with Saturn or Mars.

Read the description for any challenging aspects you may have with your Sun and determine the appropriate planetary blends and affirmations for these aspects. Start by working with the one that feels most relevant to you at this time. Then work through the others in the order of importance as outlined above. Try working with each one for a week to a month or until you feel that the energy of that challenging aspect has shifted and become more integrated.

After working through the challenging aspects to the Sun, work through the ones with your Moon in the same sequence as outlined for the Sun above.

3. WORKING WITH THE SUPPORTIVE ASPECTS
    TO YOUR SUN OR MOON

Working with the supportive aspects to your Sun or Moon from your chart will help you to identify and take hold of the supportive opportunities as they arise in your daily life. Using affirmations will help you embrace your natural talents and gifts from the universe and incorporate their expression with your Sun and Moon signs. Use the essential oils on the acupuncture points that relate to the planet in a challenging aspect, your natal Sun or Moon, or your Sun or Moon sign. Alternatively, you can apply the oils to the soles of your feet or spine.

Use the planetary blends for the supportive aspects to your Sun first and then use the ones with your Moon. Work with the oils and affirmations to more fully integrate these aspects of yourself.

In general, a conjunction or trine indicates a gift or strength that comes naturally for you. Use the appropriate planetary blend with your Sun or Moon luminary blend to strengthen your consciousness of this quality and how you express this in your life. Sextiles are strengths that you are likely to be more aware of, and you can use the appropriate planetary blends to further enhance these gifts in your life.

4. HARMONIZING WITH SEASONAL
    AND LUNAR CYCLES

Use the Transiting Sun Luminary Blend and Transiting Moon Luminary Blend to support you in attuning to the changes in the year by finding balance with the seasonal and lunar cycles. By staying in tune with the shifting rhythms and energies across the year, aligning with your true self and expressing your highest potential becomes easier.

If there is a seasonal change that is stressful for you, use the Transiting Sun Luminary Blend during that time.

Use the Transiting Moon Luminary Blend for a few days during a challenging time of a lunar cycle. Often, people are at ease with the energy of the lunar cycle that they were born into but struggle with the phase in the cycle that holds different energy. For example, if you were born at the time of the New Moon, you may feel comfortable during the time of the waxing Moon and have more difficulties with the waning part of the lunar cycle.

Use affirmations during the season or months of the year and the days of the lunar cycle you find challenging. Use the appropriate oils on any of the acupuncture points that relate to the transiting Sun or Moon, or you can apply the oils to your spine or third eye.

Optional Assessment of Aspects to Your Sun and Moon

If you are new to astrology, you may find it helpful to analyze your natal chart to determine the aspects with the strongest influences affecting your Sun and Moon signs. Using the lists below, you can assign point values to aspects in your chart and focus on the areas with the highest point values.

Sun in the sign of:

_____ (this is your Sun Sign Blend)

Moon in the sign of:

_____ (this is your Moon Sign Blend)

Assign each of the astrological aspects a point value from the list below.

For challenging aspects to the Sun or Moon use these point values:

Mars = 1   Saturn = 2   Uranus = 3
                      Chiron = 2   Neptune = 3
                                              Pluto = 3

CHALLENGING ASPECTS TO YOUR SUN:

List the planets that are in challenging aspects to your Sun. Start with the ones that have the highest point value first and work with them in the order of the most challenging aspects as shown below:
Square your Sun (within 80 to 100 degrees):

_____

Opposition to your Sun (170-190 degrees):

_____

Conjunction with your Sun (within 10 degrees):

_____

CHALLENGING ASPECTS TO YOUR MOON:

List the planets that are in challenging aspects to your Moon. Start with the ones with the highest point value first and work with them in the order of the most challenging aspects as shown below:
Square your Moon (within 80 to 100 degrees):

_____

Opposition your Moon (within 170 to 190 degrees):

_____

Conjunction with your Moon (within 10 degrees):

_____

For supportive aspects to the Sun or Moon use these point values:

Mercury = 1	Jupiter = 2	Uranus = 3
Venus = 1	Saturn = 2	Neptune = 3
Mars = 1	Chiron = 2	Pluto = 3

SUPPORTIVE ASPECTS TO YOUR SUN:

List the planets that are in supportive aspects to your Sun, then work with them in order of importance by numerical value and the strength of the supportive aspect as listed below:

Conjunctions with your Sun (within 10 degrees):

(use Mercury, Venus or Jupiter only)

_____

Trine with your Sun (within 110 to 130 degrees):

_____

Sextile with your Sun (within 50 to 70 degrees):

_____

SUPPORTIVE ASPECTS TO YOUR MOON:

List the planets that are in supportive aspects to your Moon, then work with them in order of importance by numerical value and the strength of the supportive aspect as listed below:

Conjunctions with your Moon: (within 10 degrees):

(use Mercury, Venus or Jupiter only)

_____

Trine with your Moon (within 110 to 130 degrees):

_____

Sextile with your Moon (within 50 to 70 degrees):

_____

Example:

As an example of how to work with the oils to support the Sun and Moon signs, we will look at Oprah Winfrey's chart. These are the steps that she might take in working with the oil blends and affirmations to enhance the energies of her Sun and Moon and to raise her vibrational level:

1. Supporting her Sun sign: Oprah would use the Aquarius Sign Blend since this is her Sun sign. She might use this oil blend with the affirmations for one month.

2. Supporting her Moon sign: Oprah's Moon is in the sign of Sagittarius, so she could use this sign blend for the second month to connect with and support the energies of her Moon.

3. The most challenging aspect that Oprah has with her Sun is the square with Saturn. She could use the sign blends for her Sun and Saturn (Aquarius and Scorpio) or the planetary blend for Saturn to address blocks that she has with this aspect. Working with this challenging aspect for a month would help her to clear inner blocks or conflicts and to integrate the inner strength that Saturn can offer to her Sun.

4. The most supportive aspect she has with her Sun is the trine with Jupiter, so she might want to use the sign blends for her Sun and Jupiter (Aquarius and Gemini) or the planetary blend for Jupiter for a month, to deepen her sense of faith and the self-confidence that this aspect represents.

5. Oprah does not have any challenging aspects to her Moon, so she might want to work next with the supportive aspect she has with Venus in a sextile to her Moon, by using the Venus

planetary blend or using the sign blends for her Moon and Venus (Sagittarius and Aquarius). Using these oil blends would further enhance her sensitivity and gifts in relating to others.

6.   Then Oprah might want to work with either the transiting Sun or Moon blends or with a planetary blend to address a challenging issue in her life. For example, if she felt like her energy was low, she might work with the Mars planetary blend to support her energy level.

Conclusion:

The protocols above are guidelines for how you can use the oil blends to strengthen being in your true self, living at your highest potential, and working through blocks or challenges as well as enhancing your strengths and gifts. After working with these guidelines, use your intuition to explore what oil blends and planetary energies will be most helpful for you at any given time. Working with the oil blends and affirmations as well as the archetypal energies of the Sun, Moon, and planets in your chart will deepen your understanding of yourself and increase your level of consciousness and vibrational level.

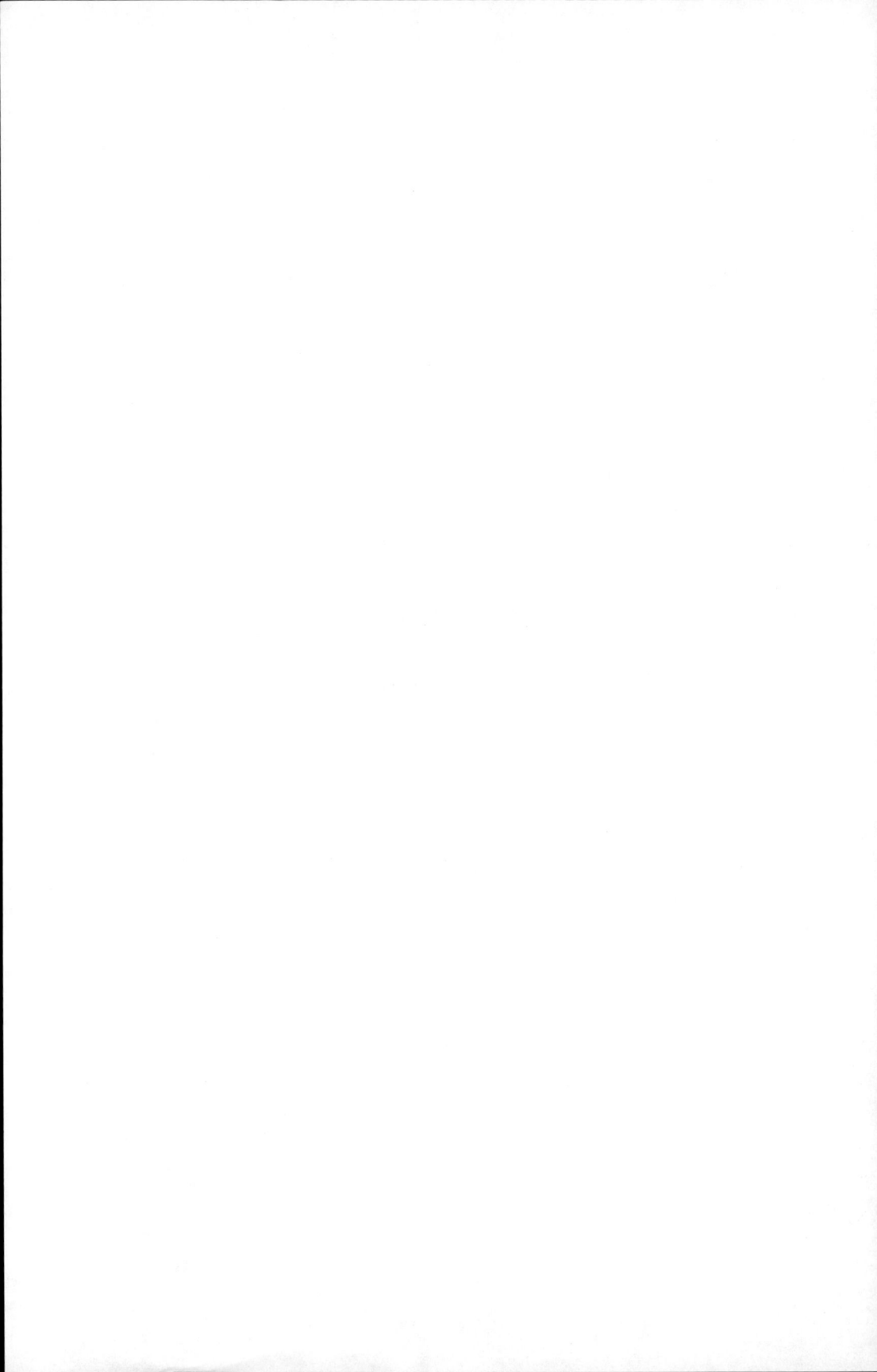

Archetypes of the Planets

U nderstanding the planetary archetypes and essential oil blends will guide you in better understanding the planets' energies in relationship with your Sun and Moon, and how you can work with those essential oil blends to support your sense of self and emotional well-being and enhance those aspects of your life.

The Mercury Archetype

The Energy of the Planet Mercury and the Stomach Meridian

Mercury is the planet closest to the Sun; it is never more than 28 degrees from the Sun in the birth chart. Mercury is also the smallest planet in our solar system. The ancient myths and understandings of Mercury are that it is the messenger, moving between the worlds. For us on the Earth, as we watch the movement of this planet, it appears to move in and out of the beams of the Sun. It is rarely visible except when it is furthest from the Sun, at which times it can be seen just before sunrise or after sunset depending on its position before or after the Sun.

The deeper meaning of Mercury relates to how we connect with the Divine Source and the light of wisdom, and how we bring that connection into our lives. Mercury also reflects the archetype of the magician, with its ability to move between the worlds and between the realm of the visible and the invisible. It is also associated with alchemy and the unification of polarities and especially of yin and yang, the feminine and masculine energies. In this way, Mercury was seen in mythology as androgynous. In addition, this planet is associated with the caduceus, which is the symbol for medicine and healing.

In your birth chart, by where it resides by sign and house and in its aspects with other planets, Mercury shows how you think and how you communicate with others. It can indicate whether you are more left-brained or right-brained, and it can highlight your strengths and weaknesses in learning and in sharing what you know with others. Mercury also indicates how you take in the light and wisdom of the Sun and allow those energies to inform you and flow through you.

When Mercury is in retrograde, as it is about three times a year for about three weeks, it indicates a period of more introspective and reflective thinking rather than more active, linear, or analytical ways of thinking and communicating. Mercury in retrograde is a time for meditation and contemplation rather than outward focus and busyness.

Mercury is the ruler of two signs: Gemini and Virgo. In Gemini, it reflects more left-brained, analytical ways of thinking and communicating. If your Mercury is in Gemini, you most likely love to learn, to take in new information, and make connections with others. If your Mercury is in Gemini, you are apt to be an excellent communicator who enjoys being in conversations with others. If your Mercury is in Virgo (symbolized as the Harvest Goddess), you may be left-brained and a detail-oriented thinker with gifts in analyzing and organizing information and in using it with discernment, "separating the wheat from the chaff."

In other signs, Mercury reflects different styles of thinking and processing information. For example, in Sagittarius, Mercury exhibits a more right-brained, integrative way of thinking. It is less focused on taking in and accumulating knowledge and is more about seeking wisdom with a longing to understand the deeper meaning of life.

If your Mercury has beneficial aspects, you may be clear in your thinking and comfortable in communicating with others. You are likely to have confidence in your intellect and enjoy learning.

If you have challenging aspects to Mercury, you may have learning difficulties, doubt your intellectual abilities, or feel that it is hard to express your thoughts. You may be self-critical or find yourself caught in obsessive thinking or anxious rumination.

In Western astrology, Mercury in Gemini is physically associated with the two hemispheres of the brain as well as the autonomic nervous system. Mercury in Virgo is associated with the digestive system. Virgo relates to the ways in which we discern what is of value to us, and to how we assimilate food in our digestive systems, particularly the intestines. Think about how often getting caught up in anxious thoughts affects your digestive system.

In Chinese medicine, Mercury corresponds to the stomach meridian. It is the only yang meridian that travels on the front of the body with the yin meridians and has yin qualities. The stomach meridian is also the only meridian that travels from the front of the body to the forehead. It accesses the frontal lobe where we intellectually process thoughts and influences every aspect associated with digestion through its interactions with and relationships to the other yang meridians.

The Harmonizing Essence of the Mercury Planetary Blend

The Mercury Planetary Blend (also known as the Stomach Meridian Balancing Blend) consists of 50% grapefruit (*Citrus x paradisi*), 25% lime (*Citrus aurantifolia*), and 25% spearmint (*Mentha spicata*). Because this blend stimulates the mind and body, the ideal time to use it is in the morning and early afternoon. The blood thinning properties of grapefruit balance the blood thickening properties of lime, thereby creating the perfect balance for blood flow and circulation. Spearmint soothes and stimulates at the same time to support mental clarity. If your essential oil manufacturer and FDA approve these oils for internal use, add a few drops to a glass of water first thing in the morning, with breakfast, and again with lunch to support healthy digestion. Applying a few drops to the sole of each foot can help you put ideas and thoughts into action.

In Chinese medicine, all medicinal substances have an energetic direction. The three essential oils in the Mercury Planetary Blend are energetically down-bearing, which can help put ideas into action. The stomach meridian easily becomes stagnant, because continually moving food down through the digestive tract can be challenging at times. If you have strong Mercury influences in your chart, you may get ideas stuck in your head and find it challenging to carry out those ideas. Energetically the Mercury Planetary Blend promotes balance between the flow of ideas and thoughts and the implementation of creative solutions.

The stomach meridian begins at the lower eyelid and travels down to the corner of the mouth, then along the jaw, in front of the ear, up to the outer edge of the forehead, then down again, passing through the thyroid area and the front of the body. The stomach meridian has the most influence over the jaw joint. If you have challenging aspects to Mercury, you may find yourself holding stress in your jaw or grinding your teeth. Aiding in the transformation of ideas into action, the Mercury Planetary Blend can focus your highly active mental energy.

How to Use the Mercury Planetary Blend

One of the important acupuncture points on the stomach meridian is Celestial Pivot, also known as *Tian Shu*, Stomach 25, or ST-25. Celestial Pivot is found about two inches on either side of the umbilicus (belly button) and is the alarm point of its paired meridian, the large intestine. Any disharmony between the stomach and large intestine meridians, or Venus and Mercury, will cause tenderness at Celestial Pivot. *Tian Shu* is the ancient name of the center star in the Big Dipper representing the pivoting point of the Dipper. The three stars that make up the handle represent divine energy or celestial *qi*.

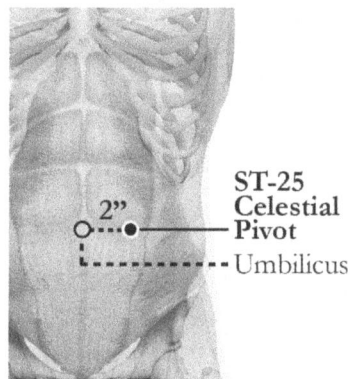

The three stars that make up the bowl represent the earthly *qi* or physical form.[2]

Applying the Mercury Planetary Blend to Celestial Pivot in a clockwise motion promotes balance between the upper and lower body, between ideas and action, and between right and left brain activity. Celestial Pivot can reset the digestive system and promote a steady flow of energy and movement in the processing of ideas into action. Applying the Mercury Planetary Blend to Celestial Pivot in a counterclockwise motion slows down the digestive process and mental activity when needed. Celestial Pivot encourages living a balanced life and harmonizing mental activity with physical activity.

Mercury Planetary Affirmations:	I learn and think with ease.
	I express myself clearly.
	I move between the worlds and feel the magic of life.

The Venus Archetype

The Energy of Venus as a Morning and Evening Star

Venus appears in the sky as an evening star for nine months out of the year, then disappears from view for a number of days. Then she emerges as a morning star for nine months. When she disappears from view again, it is for a longer period of about three

[2] Andrew Ellis, Nigel Wiseman, and Ken Boss, *Grasping the Wind* (Brookline: Paradigm Publications, 1989), 79.

months. And then the cycle starts over again. The complete cycle takes 584 days. In her movement, Venus is never more than 48 degrees from the Sun. Venus is in a dance with the Earth and the Sun, showing us how to be in relationship with Spirit, with ourselves, and with each other.

Venus moves through five cycles (as morning star and evening star) across a period of eight years before returning to her original location in relationship with the Sun and the Earth. When viewed in motion, this dance of Venus with the Sun around the Earth creates a pentacle or five-pointed star. In this way, the numbers 5, 8, and 13 are sacred to Venus and represent the energy of the Sacred Feminine. Plants with five-petaled flowers are often associated with Venus and are regarded as healing in nature.

The energies of Venus vary depending on the phase she is in. When in the evening star phase, Venus is more reflective and yin in nature. If your Venus is in this phase in your birth chart, then you may radiate an enjoyment of relationships and an ease in how you position yourself in the world. When in the morning star phase, Venus is more active, more yang, and more externally focused. If Venus is in this phase in your birth chart, you may need to interact with the world and others in an effort to learn more about yourself and about how to be in relationships. Relationships may mirror back aspects of yourself that you are striving to be more aware of and integrate.

When Venus is not visible because she is between the Sun and the Earth (in the "inferior" conjunction), she is focused on dealing with challenges in relationships. If you have this placement in your chart, you may learn lessons through difficult relationship experiences and have to face unintegrated or shadow aspects of yourself. When Venus is not visible for the longer three-month period when she circles around the back side of the Sun (in the "superior" conjunction), she carries more of the energy of needing time to be introspective, to be in relationship with yourself, to meditate and connect with Spirit, and to reflect on what you take in from your interactions with others and from integrating the light and shadow parts of yourself.

To find which phase of the Venus cycle you were born into, locate the Sun in your chart. Then move around the wheel clockwise until you locate Venus. If Venus is ahead of the Sun, then she is a morning star, rising in the east before sunrise. If she is trailing the Sun, then she is an evening star, visible low in the western sky after sunset. If Venus is within 13 degrees of the Sun, she is invisible. If Venus is in conjunction with the Sun in your birth chart and is retrograde, you were born when Venus was between the Sun and the Earth (inferior conjunction). If Venus is beside the Sun and is moving in a direct manner, then you were born when Venus was moving behind the Sun and farthest from Earth (superior conjunction).

Venus is the ruler of the signs Taurus and Libra. If your Venus is in Taurus (an earth sign), it usually means that you are grounded and have a good sense of self-worth. You likely value physical and financial security and stability. Venus in Taurus also reflects a love of beauty in a tangible and sensual way. If your Venus is in Libra, you are more focused on one-on-one relationships with others. In this sign, Venus values harmony and the ability to balance your needs with those of others. In that Libra is an air sign, the enjoyment of beauty is more intellectual and analytical. For example, with Venus in Libra, you may enjoy going to art museums as opposed to doing pottery or cooking (as with Venus in Taurus).

Where Venus resides in your birth chart by sign and house shows what you value and what you need in your relationships. Venus represents both your relationships and your internal values and external resources (including finances).

If you have beneficial aspects to Venus, you may engage easily with others and enjoy your relationships. You may also have a good sense of your self-worth and be at ease with the physical and financial resources in your life. If you have challenging aspects to Venus, you may have difficulties in relationships, struggle with your sense of self-worth, or have financial challenges.

In Western astrology, Venus is physically associated with the assimilation of sugar, with insulin, and with the senses. It relates to how you experience life in a sensual way, enjoy beauty, and take in the sweetness of life.

In Chinese medicine, Venus corresponds with the large intestine meridian in its morning star phase and with the urinary bladder meridian in its evening star phase.

Venus as a Morning Star and the Large Intestine Meridian

The Large Intestine Meridian Balancing Blend relates to Venus as a morning star, whose associated meridian rules the hours of 7 a.m. to 9 a.m. As a yang meridian, the large intestine meridian guides you through change in how to let go and how to make decisions to move forward in your life. It also influences how you internalize the world around you and how you nourish your body, mind, and spirit. The large intestine meridian controls the lower sinuses and provides energy and nutrients. Energy production depends on B vitamin absorption, which occurs in the large intestine, and sugar or carbohydrate processing, which directly impacts the healthy bacterial flora in the colon. Energy production and B vitamins are essential for the heart and cardiovascular system, illustrating the close connection Venus has to the natal Sun. The large intestine meridian controls the digestive function of the immune system found in mucous secretions called immunoglobulin A (IgA or sIgA). The consumption of carbohydrates and sugars in diets creates inflammation in the large intestine and negatively impact IgA.

Stagnation most often affects the large intestine meridian creating both blocked energy and slow metabolism. When inflammation occurs in the colon or the bacterial flora are out of balance, stiffness and discomfort can occur in the lower back while sleeping, and you may feel worse upon waking in the morning. The physical signs of stagnation, including constipation, weight gain, and congestion, correspond with the emotions of feeling blocked, unable to enjoy life to the fullest, and even feeling trapped in unhealthy situations. Supporting the large intestine meridian will help you start your day on a positive note with direction and clarity.

The Harmonizing Essence of the Venus Morning Star Blend

The planetary blend for Venus as a morning star (also known as the Large Intestine Meridian Balancing Blend) consists of 50% palmarosa (*Cymbopogon martinii*), 25% lemongrass (*Cymbopogon citratus*), and 25% citronella (*Cymbopogon nardus*). All three of these plants are from gramineae species of grasses, which support the body's healthy bacterial flora. Supporting these beneficial bacteria will offset diets high in sugar, carbohydrates, and alcohol.

Palmarosa, known as Turkish rose, preserves beauty, benefits the skin, promotes anti-aging, and carries a high vibration similar to rose, but for a fraction of the cost. Citronella and lemongrass uplift and energize while balancing the relaxing and calming properties of palmarosa. Citronella and lemongrass are commonly used to keep pests (insects and nonbeneficial people) away while providing a cleansing and refreshing aroma.

The Venus Morning Star blend encourages experiencing the sweetness of life with balance and at a steady pace. The beneficial properties of palmarosa for the skin offset the irritating properties of citronella and lemongrass. However, this blend should be diluted 50/50 if you have sensitive skin or are using it daily. Applying this blend to the soles of the feet or diffusing it in the morning are the best uses for this blend undiluted.

How to Use the Venus Morning Star Blend

One of the best-known points in Chinese medicine is Union Valley, also known as *He Gu*, Large Intestine 4, or LI-4. As one of the "Four Gates," Union Valley both protects the borders of the body and allows energy to enter the meridian system. When combined with Great Surge (Liver 3, LV-3), Union Valley point balances and supports the entire meridian system. Union Valley is one of the ancient "eleven heavenly star points" and is the command point for the face and mouth. This point commonly treats headaches, cold or flu symptoms, swelling of the face, and the inability to speak. Union Valley has an analgesic effect on the brain when vigorously massaged to help relieve pain anywhere in the body. Union Valley strongly promotes uterine contractions and is avoided during pregnancy until the 39th and 40th weeks to encourage the labor process.

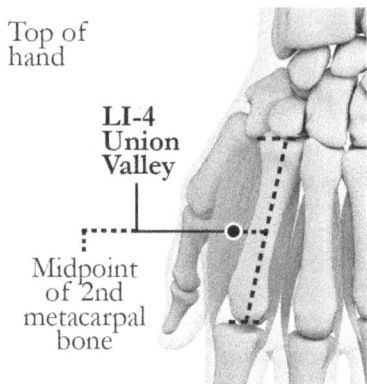

Top of hand

LI-4 Union Valley

Midpoint of 2nd metacarpal bone

Union Valley is found a variety of ways. One method locates this point on the topside or dorsum of the hand, between the first finger and the thumb, at the midpoint of the second metacarpal bone. Union Valley means mountain, and with the thumb and fingers held tightly, the point is found at the highest juncture of the muscle between the thumb and first finger. An alternative name for this point is Tiger's Mouth, because of the special ability of thumb and forefinger to open widely and the special movement of the thumb.[3] Massaging the diluted Venus morning star blend into the Union Valley point clockwise supports adding energy into the body, releasing stuck emotions, and relieving pain. Massaging the diluted blend counterclockwise triggers the immune system to fight off viruses and bacteria. Massaging the blend into this point back and forth in all directions is best for promoting labor.

Another beneficial point on the large intestine meridian is Arm Three Li, also known as Large Intestine 10, or LI-10. *Li*, a Chinese unit of measurement that is one-third of a mile, refers to regulating the three distinct levels of the body similar to Union Valley's ability to regulate the entire meridian system. Arm Three

[3]Andrew Ellis, Nigel Wiseman, and Ken Boss, *Grasping the Wind* (Brookline: Paradigm Publications, 1989), 39-40.

Li is found on the forearm, close to the elbow, at the highest point in the muscle when the arm is tightly bent and lying across the chest. Arm Three Li stores the body's memories of allergies and sensitivities and is tender on

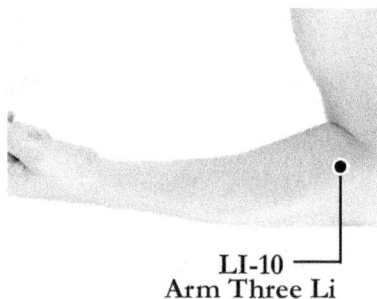

LI-10
Arm Three Li

most people. Massaging the diluted Venus Morning Star Blend clockwise into this area in the morning can help release the body's memory of allergies and sensitivities. Arm Three Li releases emotional blockages and feelings of carrying the weight of the world on our shoulders. The releasing nature of this point helps relieve shoulder discomfort and constipation. Also, Arm Three Li is a safe alternative to Union Valley during pregnancy because of Union Valley's releasing nature.

Always dilute the Venus Morning Star blend when applying to the above acupuncture points. This blend contains lemongrass, which can irritate sensitive and sun-damaged skin. The standard dilution is 50/50 with a carrier oil, however, if you have sensitive or sun-damaged skin, dilute 25/75 with a carrier oil. You can use this blend undiluted in a diffuser or on the soles of the feet. The Venus Morning Star affirmations can enhance this blend for both diffusing and topical application.

Venus Morning Star Affirmations:

I savor the sweetness of life.

I know my worth and value myself.

I relate to others from a centered place.

Venus as an Evening Star and the Urinary Bladder Meridian

The Urinary Bladder Meridian Balancing Blend relates to Venus as an evening star, whose associated meridian rules the hours of 3 p.m. to 5 p.m. The urinary bladder meridian influences how you take in the world and externalize your emotions. It controls the central nervous system and sensory perception, which influences the processing of information and assigns meaning to what happened. These functions are closely related to the hypothalamus and governing vessel and again illustrate the close relationship Venus has to the natal Sun. This is the largest meridian in the body, and it functions as a healthy boundary relative to your immediate environment.

A balanced urinary bladder meridian allows for flexibility in dealing with others and effectiveness in communication, which are the keys to lasting relationships. Gentleness with others and yourself can soften challenging aspects to Venus as an evening star. With age and increased responsibility, supporting your urinary bladder meridian will help keep your back strong and flexible.

Short-term imbalances in the urinary bladder meridian correspond with both a strained back and strained relationships. If imbalances are long-term, then posture becomes compromised, and relationships can feel chronically strained and even unhealthy. Poor posture negatively impacts how information affects the nervous system. The best place to apply the Evening Star Venus Blend is along the spine, which requires help from someone to reach the entire back, another example of why relationships are important.

The Harmonizing Essence of the Venus Evening Star Blend

The planetary blend for Venus as an evening star (also known as the Urinary Bladder Meridian Balancing Blend) consists of 50% marjoram (*Origanum majorana*), 25% cedarwood (*Cedrus atlantica*), and 25% copaiba (copal: *Copaifera reticulate* or *Copaifera L. genus*). This blend encourages healthy relationships by supporting appropriate boundaries, promoting flexibility, adapting to changing situations, and releasing irritating habits. These three oils together balance the nervous system, helping you adapt to any situation and challenge you may find yourself in.

Marjoram reduces stress hormones, promotes relaxation, and releases stored stress from tight or knotted muscles. Copaiba stimulates the body and mind to take action while creating healthy boundaries for self-preservation. Copaiba is a resin and, in general, trees make resin to heal wounds, sealing the site of injury to keep pathogens out and ensuring the tree's longevity. Indigenous cultures in South and Central America use copaiba in ceremony to connect with the spirit world.

Cedarwood is an adaptogenic essential oil, which means it can intuitively change the healing properties based on your immediate needs. For example, cedarwood in the morning promotes healthy cortisol levels for energy production and increased focus. In the evening, cedarwood promotes healthy melatonin levels for sleep and relaxation. Cedarwood's ability to adapt to the body's changing needs occurs by supporting the nervous system and the hypothalamus. Marjoram directs healing nutrients to the muscles, and copaiba directs healing nutrients to the bones and brain. Together they address every level in the body's nervous system with the ability to adapt to where the healing energy is needed.

How to Use the Venus Evening Star Blend

The urinary bladder meridian runs along the spinal nerves and has the most acupuncture points of any meridian. Because of this, it includes many important and regularly used acupuncture points and applying the Venus Evening Star Bend along the entire spine will balance these important neurological points. The spirit points that support balanced relationships, and a connection to your higher self, include Heaven's Pillar, Kunlun Mountains, and Extending Vessel.

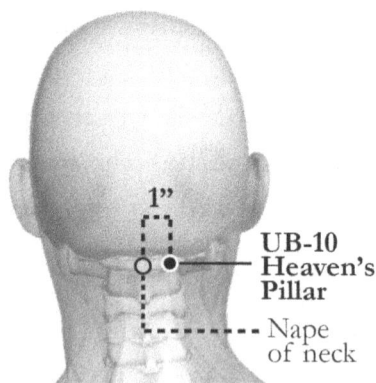

Heaven's Pillar, also known as *Tian Zhu*, Urinary Bladder 10, UB-10, or BL-10, is found at the hairline on the back of the neck about one inch on both sides from the center of the spine, known as the nape of the neck. Heaven's Pillar is a special "Window of Heaven" point, which corrects the flow of energy in the body when the yin (natal Moon) and yang (natal Sun) are in conflict with each other. If your natal Sun and Moon are in a challenging aspect to one another, this point can help harmonize and integrate these energies. Heaven's Pillar connects the hypothalamus with the pituitary gland and creates the foundation for the endocrine system and all of your hormones. This point becomes tender when the hypothalamus-pituitary connection is weak, or the hormones are out of balance. Apply the Venus Evening Star Blend across the back of the neck, connecting Heaven's Pillar on each side of the body to balance the yin and yang of the body and strengthen your connection with your higher-self, spirit guides, universal source, or God, depending on your belief system.

Kunlun Mountains, known as Urinary Bladder 60, UB-60, or BL-60, is found on the outside of the anklebone in a depression between the anklebone (lateral malleolus) and the Achilles tendon. The Kunlun Mountains are one of the largest mountain ranges in China. Legend states

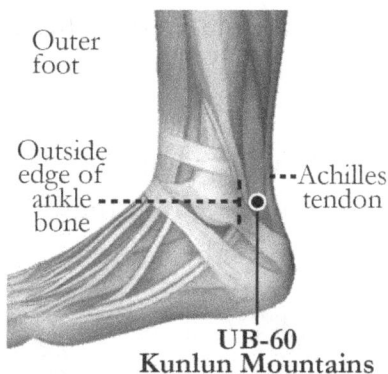

Outer foot

Outside edge of ankle bone

Achilles tendon

UB-60
Kunlun Mountains

that the tallest peak, Kunlun Mountain, is where the spirit transitions from Heaven to Earth. Kunlun is one of the twelve Heavenly Star Points and has a special connection with Heaven's Pillar; they are commonly used together to harmonize the body, mind, and spirit. Apply the Venus Evening Star Blend in a clockwise motion at this point to strengthen your body, mind, and spirit connection.

Extending Vessel, known as *Shen Mai*, Urinary Bladder 62, UB-62, or BL-62, is found about half an inch below the outside of the anklebone in a depression below the peroneal tendons. Extending Vessel accesses one of the eight extra vessels called the Yang Motility Vessel and pairs it with

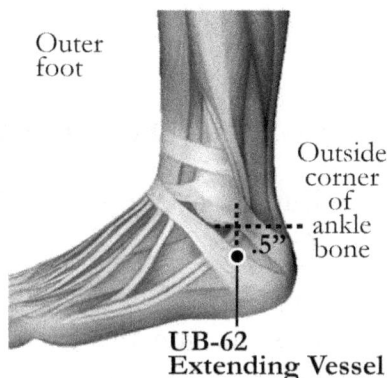

Outer foot

Outside corner of ankle bone

.5"

UB-62
Extending Vessel

the governing vessel, which represents the natal Sun. The Yang

Motility Vessel influences your ability to move forward and can help give direction on the next steps to take on your spiritual path. Extending Vessel is one of the thirteen ghost points used to strengthen your *shen* or spirit. Apply the Venus Evening Star Blend in a clockwise motion to Extending Vessel when you need direction from your higher self or spirit guides on the next steps to take in life.

The Venus Evening Star blend only requires dilution if you have sensitive skin, are using this blend long-term, or have short hair that exposes the hairline at the back of the neck.

Venus Evening Star Affirmations:	I honor my feelings and needs and those of others.
	I value balance and harmony in life and in my relationships.
	I reflect on my decisions and act in accordance with my values.

The Mars Archetype

The Energy of the Planet Mars and Lung Meridian

Mars is the first planet whose orbit is outside of our Earth orbit. It circles the Sun in 687 days and takes twenty-six months to complete its full cycle. Mars is the first planet out from the Sun that can be visible anywhere in the sky as it orbits around the Earth. It is red in color and glows most brightly when it is opposite the Sun in the sky.

In its meaning, Mars reflects how we move out into the world. Mars, by sign and house in astrology charts, gives information about our energy, how we act and how we assert ourselves. Archetypally, it reflects our path of individuation and how we each are progressing on our own hero's journey of growth and exploration in this lifetime.

If your Mars is in a cardinal sign, you are quick to take action and are likely to be more of a risk-taker, comfortable with initiating new projects or moving in new directions. If your Mars is in a fixed sign, you may be more willing to persevere in your focus in work or on a project, following through to completion. If in a mutable sign, you are more adaptable and comfortable shifting direction, making changes when needed.

In earth signs with Mars, you may be focused on taking action and seeing clear, tangible results. In a fire sign, you enjoy stimulation, challenges, and being inspired as well as wanting to express yourself in creative ways. In air signs, you may reflect on how you want to act and think things through before moving in a new direction. You may have an active mind and enjoy mental activity. If in a water sign, your actions are apt to be influenced by your moods and emotions, and you are likely to act in a sensitive way, considering the consequences of your actions on others.

Mars is the ruler of the sign of Aries. In Aries, it reflects the need to act, to take initiative, and to explore the world. Aries is a cardinal fire sign, and Mars in this sign indicates a tendency to be impulsive or quick to act, sometimes not thinking through the consequences of actions. It can also manifest in a fiery nature and being quick to anger, but the anger dissipates just as rapidly as it arises. Aries also indicates leadership qualities and a strong will or tendency to be "head-strong."

In traditional astrology, Mars is also the ruler of Scorpio. In this fixed water sign, Mars shows a tendency to be passionate as well as a possible tendency to brood, to hold on to anger or resentments and to repress anger until it may explode or be acted out in a destructive way.

With supportive or beneficial aspects to Mars in your birth chart, you may have strong energy and be comfortable with taking action and being assertive. You are generally balanced and thoughtful in how you act and think through the consequences of your actions. You are effective in how you move through life. You are also likely to be slow to anger and are able to consider how you want to express your frustration or anger with others. You may have leadership skills or be successful in how you take action in the world.

If Mars is out of balance or in challenging aspects, you may have low energy, have difficulty with motivating yourself to take action, or may be at the opposite extreme and have a tendency to be overly aggressive. Mars out of balance also reflects a tendency to either suppress your anger or express it in an unbalanced way. It may also show a pattern of impulsivity or of being accident prone.

In Western astrology, Mars is physically associated with the blood (especially red blood cells), the adrenal glands, and with physical activity and sexual expression.

In Chinese medicine, Mars corresponds to the lung meridian, which controls breathing, the skin, the immune system, energizing cells with oxygen, and your relationship to your environment. Immune weakness or autoimmune tendencies are signs that the lung meridian is out of balance. A balanced lung meridian encourages you to have healthy breathing patterns and appropriate responses to your surroundings, both physically and emotionally.

Both Mars and Pluto and their respective meridians influence the reproductive organs and sexual energy. Mars provides the sex drive and passion, while Pluto rules the reproductive organs. The lung meridian is also responsible for blood flow and oxygenating the reproductive organs.

In Chinese medicine, the heart organ governs pumping the blood, and the lung meridian governs the vessels (arteries, capillaries, and veins) that hold the blood in place. As the heart pumps, the lungs oxygenate the blood, which is the main function of red blood cells, also ruled by Mars.

The Harmonizing Essence of the Mars Planetary Blend

The planetary blend for Mars (also known as the Lung Meridian Balancing Blend) consists of 50% lavender (*Lavandula angustifolia*), 25% tea tree (*Melaleuca alternifolia*), and 25% niaouli (*Melaleuca quinquenervia*). While the two *Melaleuca* species are from the same family, their healing properties differ. Tea tree is stronger against pathogenic infections and helps with cleansing the skin and air. Niaouli contains plant-based male-type hormones, which promote tissue regeneration, and is strongest against fungus and radiation when compared to other *Melaleuca* oils. Lavender is calming, relaxing, and regenerative. Lavender's slightly phytoestrogenic properties balance niaouli's slightly phytotestosterone properties; it calms the natural aggressive properties of Mars.

The Mars Planetary Blend addresses physical irritation or trauma to the skin and emotional insults or boundary challenges. This blend is perfect for the everyday athlete, helps keep away outdoor pests, and promotes a healthy immune response to any climate. All three of the oils in the Mars Blend support a balanced immune response by helping the immune system regulate and react to different environmental stimuli. This blend softens any Mars aspect by integrating the internal struggle of inaction and over-action with self-acceptance.

How to Use the Mars Planetary Blend

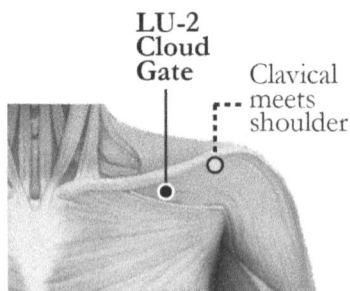

LU-2
Cloud
Gate   Clavical
           meets
           shoulder

Cloud Gate, also known as *Yun Men*, Lung 2, or LU-2 can help you start the twenty-four-hour meridian cycle (which begins with the lung meridian) on a positive and healthy note, such as starting your day on the right foot, taking the first steps of a race, or planning your day. Cloud Gate is found on the upper chest just below the lateral end of the clavicle bone in a groove that forms when you raise your arm. Because this point rests so close to the lung organ, Cloud Gate is rarely accessed with acupuncture needles and responds best to essential oils. According to the classics, "Earth's *qi* ascends as clouds; heaven's *qi* descends as rain."[4] Here Cloud Gate is the entry point for Earth's *qi* to enter and add energy into the acupuncture meridian system.

Applying a 50/50 dilution of the Mars Planetary Blend in a clockwise circle will stimulate and add energy to the meridian system. The ideal time to apply the blend to Cloud Gate is either before bed or if you wake up before 5 a.m. in the morning to synchronize with the peak time of the lung meridian.

Another important acupuncture point on the lung meridian is Broken Sequence, also known as *Lie Que*, Lung 7, or LU-7. This point is found just proximal (closer to the body) to the styloid process of the wrist. Broken Sequence is easiest to find by interlocking your thumbs in the webbing between the thumb and index finger. The index finger of the top hand should lie on the styloid process.

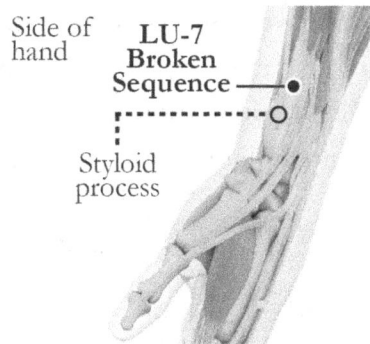

Broken Sequence is the master command point for the head and is a heavenly star point. It is highly effective in treating headaches and migraines. Broken Sequence is the access point to the conception vessel, Natal Moon, which strongly influences emotional health, reproduction, and creativity. Broken Sequence connects the lung meridian to the large intestine meridians in the twenty-four-hour meridian circulation pattern. An alternate name for this point is Child Mystery, and it is commonly used in treating children. The leading cause of harm to young children is accidents (ruled by Mars) and complications affecting the lungs such as influenza, pneumonia, and asthma.

---

[4] Andrew Ellis, Nigel Wiseman, and Ken Boss, *Grasping the Wind* (Brookline: Paradigm Publications, 1989), 25.

Another translation for Broken Sequence is "thunderhead spitting fire," which describes a challenged Mars aspect not properly handled. Mars can trigger conflicts and hot tempers when emotions are not consciously managed. The Mars Planetary Blend soothes and softens challenging aspects from Mars. Diffusing this blend at night supports the lungs while you sleep. Apply this blend directly to the soles of the feet, the back of the neck, or any area that has experienced trauma or excessive sun exposure. Dilute this blend 50/50 with a carrier oil if you have sensitive skin, are applying it to a large area, or are using it long-term. Incorporating the following affirmations with the Mars Blend application to Broken Sequence can help you focus as you contemplate appropriate actions.

Mars Planetary Affirmations:	I act in a clear and decisive manner. I assert myself with confidence. I know that I am learning and growing through all of my experiences.

The Jupiter Archetype

The Energy of the Planet Jupiter and the Pericardium Meridian

Jupiter is the largest planet in the solar system and is twice the size of all of the other planets combined. It is a gas giant whose composition is different from the terrestrial planets and is more

---

5 Andrew Ellis, Nigel Wiseman, and Ken Boss, *Grasping the Wind* (Brookline: Paradigm Publications, 1989), 30-31.

like that of a star. Jupiter has such a strong gravitational field that it pulls comets and asteroids into its orbit and, in that way, protects us here on Earth. Archetypally, the planet holds the energy of a protector, teacher, and guru.

Where Jupiter resides by sign and house in your natal chart gives information about your beliefs, your sense of optimism or faith, and your deeper understanding of life. It is associated with higher education, with learning through experience and through being exposed to other cultures (travel), as well as with integrative thinking (seeing the bigger picture).

Jupiter is the ruler of Sagittarius, a mutable fire sign. Sagittarius is the constellation close to the Milky Way that depicts the archer holding the bow and arrow. The tip of the arrow points to the black rift in the Milky Way, which is the view of the center of our galaxy from the Earth. In this way, Jupiter in Sagittarius reflects the search for Source, for the deeper meaning of life.

Jupiter carries the energy of fate and new possibilities and supports you in your endeavors. Jupiter tends to be beneficial in its aspects to other planets. When it is in balance in your chart, it reflects a sense of faith even in times of stress and a capacity to move forward through challenging times, knowing that the light comes after the darkest night.

If Jupiter is in challenging aspects in your chart, so that its supportive energy is being blocked or constricted, you may tend to get lost in details and have trouble seeing the bigger picture. It may be hard to hold onto a sense of faith or hope. You may not know what to believe, or struggle to define your view of the meaning of life. Or, at the other end of the spectrum, an out of balance Jupiter may indicate overly high ideals, rigid beliefs, or a grandiose sense of self. This may be reflected in being adventurous yet feeling scattered, like the explorer who travels the world needing to be in motion without a deeper purpose or intention.

Physically, in Western astrology, Jupiter is associated with growth, weight gain, and with the liver and kidneys.

In Chinese medicine, Jupiter relates to the pericardium meridian, which has very different functions than it does in Western medicine. The pericardium is a double-walled membrane that wraps around the heart and the large blood vessels of the heart. The pericardium protects the heart and holds it in place in the chest cavity. While the heart is the sovereign fire, the pericardium is the ministerial fire, which is in service to the heart. In Chinese medicine, the heart and pericardium meridians together direct the pituitary gland that influences all hormone activity in the body. The pericardium meridian controls the hormones that influence digestion, blood sugar regulation, and blood creation. Because of the close ties with blood, the pericardium meridian is more active in women who are having a regular menstrual cycle. Along with the heart meridian, the pericardium meridian strongly influences mental health, and specifically those conditions that cause restlessness, anxiousness, and inappropriate responses to stress. An imbalanced pericardium meridian contributes to premenstrual symptoms in menstruating women.

The Harmonizing Essence of the Jupiter Planetary Blend

The Jupiter Planetary Blend (also known as the Pericardium Meridian Balancing Blend) consists of 50% lavender (*Lavandula angustifolia*), 25% balsam fir (*Abies balsamea*), and 25% patchouli (*Pogostemon cablin*). All three of these oils relax the body, calm the mind, and soothe the spirit by cooling the blood and balancing hormones. All of these oils have properties that harmonize hormone levels to support a balanced endocrine system.

Balsam fir is a small species of the fir family and is commonly harvested as a Christmas tree in Northern America. This fir can grow to 50 or 60 feet in height and is perfectly conical in shape as it reaches for the heavens. As an evergreen conifer, a fir tree will hold its color and needles all year, representing holding on to values and a higher purpose through any climate. Patchouli dissolves environmental toxins and the buildup of excess hormones, especially stress hormones. Patchouli dispels toxic thoughts while supporting feelings of unconditional love and acceptance as it protects the heart. Lavender adapts to any situation and cools the excessive heat that easily builds up in the pericardium meridian. The Jupiter Planetary Blend has both restorative and protective properties for the body, mind, and spirit to help you weather any emotional storm.

How to Use the Jupiter Planetary Blend

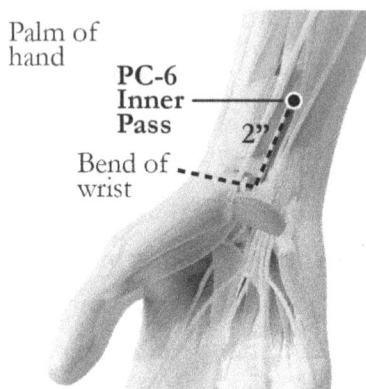

Palm of hand
PC-6
Inner Pass
2"
Bend of wrist

The acupuncture point Inner Pass, also known as *Nei Guan*, Inner Gate, Pericardium 6, or PC 6, is the access point for the yin linking vessel and the connecting point to the triple burner meridian, which relates to the planet Saturn. The yin linking vessel unites the yin meridians together to regulate the body's blood and fluids, to relax and promote restoration while sleeping, and to calm the emotions.

Inner Pass is found on the inside of the forearm, two inches proximal (closer to the body) from the wrist crease, between two larger tendons that run down the middle of the forearm. Activating Inner Pass encourages you to nourish your body, mind, and spirit with a higher vibration through high-quality food, positive internal dialogue, and staying true to your ideals. Applying the Jupiter Planetary Blend in a downward motion from Inner Pass to the wrist crease will harmonize your yin meridians, calm your emotions, and help you focus your actions while supporting strength and flexibility in the wrist.

The acupuncture point Celestial Spring, also known as *Tian Quan*, Heaven Source, Pericardium 2, or PC 2, funnels down energy from the heavens to flow here on Earth. Celestial Spring encourages the connection with your higher self to flow into daily life as an expression of your soul's purpose in this lifetime. Celestial Spring can be found on the inner arm two inches distal from the armpit fold with the arm raised. Applying the Jupiter Planetary Blend in a clockwise motion to Celestial Spring before bed can help you align with your soul's purpose and discover new ways to integrate that purpose into your daily life. Applying the Jupiter Planetary Blend to this point

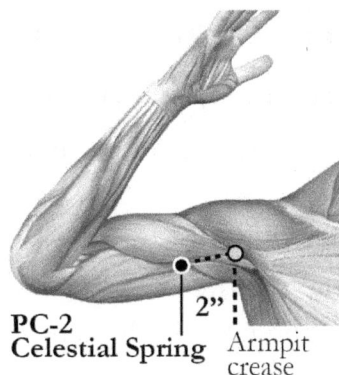

PC-2
Celestial Spring · 2" · Armpit crease

in a clockwise motion before traveling or setting out on new adventures will strengthen your connection with your guardian angels and provide protection while on your journeys.

Diffusing the Jupiter Planetary Blend during the peak time for the pericardium meridian, between the hours of 7 p.m. and 9 p.m., will harmonize the meridian and help release stressors from the day. This is the ideal time to create healthy habits promoting rest and relaxation including yin yoga, stretching, meditation, or a relaxing walk to release frustration from your day's activities.

Jupiter Planetary Affirmations:	I have faith in life and feel guided and protected. I know that life is a journey of exploration and growth. I trust in who I am and my purpose in life.

The Saturn Archetype

The Energy of the Planet Saturn and the Triple Burner Meridian

Saturn is the sixth planet from the Sun. It is a gas giant like Jupiter and is the second largest planet in our solar system. It is the last visible planet in the solar system, and so guards the threshold between our visible reality and the invisible outer solar system. Traditionally, Saturn has been associated with fears, constrictions, blocks, and what weighs us down. Where Saturn resides by sign and house may be where we encounter challenges or tests that guide us into deeper self-awareness and wisdom.

The more ancient archetypal understanding of Saturn is that it is the "god of the sweet waters," helping us move between the worlds. Saturn is the only planet that is less dense than water. It can teach us how to live our lives in a fluid way. Saturn, as the wise elder or teacher, can guide us in how to bring our deeper soul awareness into form. And it can support us in how we structure and manifest our lives here on the Earth plane, in visible reality. When we work with Saturn's deeper meaning and purpose, it brings wisdom and inner strength.

Saturn is the ruler of Capricorn. When in this sign, Saturn reflects the ability to manifest goals and to live from a deeper sense of wisdom, passion, and purpose.

Saturn in beneficial aspects to other planets tends to support those planets in bringing their energy into manifestation. Saturn can strengthen other planets and help you to persevere through times of stress. It is also grounding and stabilizing to you and in its influence on other planets.

When Saturn is in challenging aspects in your natal chart, it may reflect working the shadow side of Saturn. It may then show you where you feel blocked, constricted, constrained or controlled by others, or misunderstood. It may also reflect your own self-criticism or difficulties in seeing yourself clearly and fully valuing yourself. If Saturn is in challenging aspects with other planets, Saturn will tend to constrict the energy of that planet or delay its ability to manifest itself in your life. For example, if Saturn is squaring Venus, this may result in difficulties in relationships. However, once the right relationship is found, Saturn brings a sense of commitment and willingness to stay the course.

Physically, Saturn is associated with the bones and skeletal system and the physical structure of our bodies.

In Chinese medicine, Saturn corresponds to the triple burner meridian, which has no exact translation in Western medicine. The triple burner connects the upper third (the spirit), the middle third (the emotions), and the lower third (the physical body) to unify the three aspects of the self. In Japanese-style acupuncture, the triple burner meridian corresponds to the lymph system. The lymph system generates a few adult stem cells called hematopoietic stem cells, which are rare and hold the potential for extensive regeneration and the ability to differentiate into all blood cell types. These stem cells are the raw materials for regeneration and depend on a balanced meridian system to properly activate for healing.

The Harmonizing Essence of the Saturn Planetary Blend

The Saturn Planetary Blend (also known as the Triple Burner Meridian Balancing Blend) consists of 50% cypress (*Cupressus sempervirens*), 25% tangerine (*Citrus nobilis* or *Citrus reticulata* var. *tangerine*), and 25% grapefruit (*Citrus x paradisi*). In Chinese medicine, evergreen trees symbolize eternal life, promote anti-aging, and support the DNA. Cypress trees are one the oldest species of evergreen, dating back over 150 million years. They grow in harsh climates, including poor soil, dry conditions, and standing water. Cypress essential oil promotes circulation of the lymph system and balancing of the meridian system to support healthy activation of adult stem cells for regeneration.

Citrus essential oils are cold-pressed from the inside white part of the rind which forms the outer boundary of the fruit. Tangerine is energetically uplifting, and grapefruit is energetically down-bearing; together they promote continual flow and circulation in the body. Challenging aspects from Saturn can at times force you to work through difficult situations, and these three oils together promote the balanced forward movement for the spirit, the mind, and the body. The Saturn Planetary blend can help you move past limitations and blockages while balancing the body, mind, and spirit.

How to Use the Saturn Planetary Blend

The acupuncture point Outer Pass, also known as *Wai Guan*, Outer Gate, Triple Burner 5, or TB 5, is the access point for the yang linking vessel and the connecting point to the pericardium meridian. Outer pass unites the yang meridians to protect the body and regulate energy resources during the day. This extra vessel is responsible for adjusting the body to harsh weather patterns and abrupt changes in climate. Outer Pass is found on the outside of the forearm, one and a half inches proximal (closer to the body) from the wrist crease, in the depression between the ulnar and radial bones.

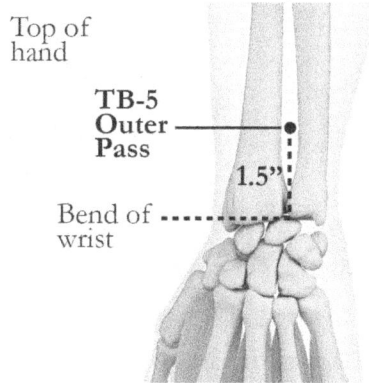

Activating Outer Pass can help you take yourself out into the world in a balanced way. Because of the two citrus oils in this blend intensify the effects of the sun, we recommend applying the Saturn Planetary Blend, diluted 50/50 with a carrier oil, to Outer Pass before going to bed or during the meridian peak time of 9 p.m. to 11 p.m. Applying the Saturn Planetary Blend in a clockwise motion will enhance the moving properties of it. Diffusing this blend or applying it full strength to the soles of the feet are other options for harmonizing Saturn in your chart. Working with the following affirmations and the Saturn Planetary Blend can help you soften the challenging aspects of Saturn and harness the beneficial ones.

Saturn Planetary Affirmations:	I grow in wisdom and am guided by Spirit. I know who I am and my purpose, and I live that daily. I manifest with ease.

The Uranus Archetype

The Energy of the Planet Uranus and the Gallbladder Meridian

Uranus is the seventh planet in the solar system and orbits beyond Saturn. It is the first of the three outermost planets; these three (Uranus, Neptune, and Pluto) are known as the transpersonal planets because they carry more generational themes in our charts and also help us gain insight and to transform by connecting us with the spiritual energies of the cosmos.

Uranus is an unusual planet in that it breaks the rules of typical planetary behavior. For example, most planets spin on an axis perpendicular to the plane of the ecliptic; but Uranus' axis is almost parallel to the ecliptic. While its south pole points almost directly at the Sun, it receives less energy from the Sun than its equatorial regions. The ways that Uranus breaks out of the usual planetary patterns parallel its archetypal meaning in our lives. Where Uranus resides, by house and sign, shows where we break free of cultural norms and conditioning to express our uniqueness. It may be where we challenge authority or "break the rules." Those of us with a strong Uranus in our charts are often rebels, reformers, pioneers, nonconformists, or we tend to be creative or make ground-breaking discoveries.

Uranus is the modern ruler of Aquarius, and in this sign, it indicates someone with strong social and humanitarian ideals. Uranus in Aquarius reflects a strong sense of fairness, openness to diversity, and concern for social justice.

In traditional astrology, however, Saturn is the ruler of Aquarius.

It represents a more traditional honoring of systems and institutions and a reluctance for change.

If your Uranus is in balance or in positive aspects to the Sun or Moon, you may be a visionary, a truth-teller, or a reformer who strives to serve a larger purpose beneficial to humanity. This connection between Uranus and the Sun or Moon also often indicates possible psychic gifts or the ability to gain insights from the "Divine Mind" through sudden flashes of knowing or through understanding the meaning of synchronicities. Uranus also fosters creativity and clarity.

If out of balance or in challenging aspects to other planets (especially the Sun or Moon), Uranus may indicate that you are a person who is arrogant, disruptive, unpredictable, or fearful of change.

Physically, Uranus is associated with neural activity as well as the assimilation of oxygen.

In Chinese medicine, Uranus corresponds to the gallbladder meridian. The emotion associated with the gallbladder meridian is gall or audacity. When in balance, gall means the willingness to take bold risks; when out of balance, gall means rude or disrespectful behavior. The gallbladder is responsible for properly digesting fats, which the brain and nervous system depend on to function. Nerves have a myelin sheath, which looks like the plastic covering on an electrical wire that conducts the nerve impulses. The body repairs the myelin sheath using properly digested healthy fats.

Hydrogenated fats and genetically modified foods, such as GMO corn used to make vegetable or corn oil, easily compromise the gallbladder meridian. The gallbladder meridian pathway includes the temples and sides of the head and is responsible for stress and tension headaches. Choosing high-quality fats and diets higher in omega-3 fats from fish, olive, avocado, and walnut oils can help support your gallbladder meridian.

The gallbladder meridian corresponds to connective tissue, including tendons, ligaments, and the myofascial layer which allows the bones and muscles to glide on top of each other. The connective tissues are responsible for fluid movement, and this corresponds to fluid thoughts and emotions. Keeping the gallbladder meridian balanced promotes free thinking and a willingness to change direction.

The Harmonizing Essence of the Uranus Planetary Blend

The Uranus Planetary Blend (also known as the Gallbladder Meridian Balancing Blend) consists of 50% marjoram (*Origanum majorana*), 25% rosemary (*Rosmarinus officianalis*), and 25% tangerine (*Citrus nobilis* or *Citrus reticulata* var. *tangerine*). Marjoram targets the connective tissue layer and the muscles of the body. Marjoram simultaneously increases strength in the connective tissue and muscles while relaxing them. Rosemary is beneficial for any long-term or chronic imbalance in the body or the spirit, and it can help overcome hidden factors holding back spiritual development. Tangerine strongly uplifts the mood and energizes the body. This blend provides the strength and flexibility to understand and transform outdated concepts that are holding you back, whether it be societal repression, family constraints, or self-limiting ideas.

Marjoram is calming, regulates blood pressure, and encourages a relaxed but robust approach to life. Rosemary is stimulating and energizing to help you take action. However, rosemary essential oil can increase blood pressure if you have high blood pressure or a family history of hypertension. Spearmint essential oil is the recommended substitute for rosemary due to its stimulating and cleansing properties. Marjoram naturally balances rosemary if you have normal or lower blood pressure.

How to Use the Uranus Planetary Blend

The gallbladder meridian connects the front and back sides of the body and travels from the side of the head or temple area, down along the side of the body to the ankle and fourth toe. The gallbladder meridian links the surface layers of the body, which include the immune system, to the deeper layers of the body, which include the bones and internal organs. The gallbladder meridian integrates the core of who you are with your community or environment. Two acupuncture points found on the gallbladder meridian can address both challenging and beneficial aspects of Uranus. Celestial Hub, found above the apex of the ear, can help you process new ideas, and Hill Ruins found on the outside of the ankle can help take action and implement the new ideas.

The acupuncture point Celestial Hub, also known as *Tian Chong*, Celestial Surge, Celestial Crossroads, Heavenly Rushing, Gallbladder 9, or GB-9, is found one inch above the top of the outer ear. Celestial Hub sits over the temporal lobe of the brain,

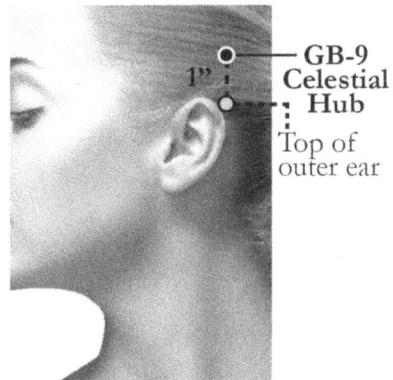

GB-9
Celestial
Hub
Top of
outer ear
1"

which processes listening and comprehension of words and ideas. Celestial Hub is the meeting point of the gallbladder and urinary bladder meridians, and several sources state that the point found a half-inch behind or posterior to it, GB-8, which is the meeting point of all the yang meridians, is really Celestial Hub.

Because of the closeness of these two points, when you apply the Uranus Planetary Blend in this area you will also harmonize both points and all the yang meridians of the body. Temporal headaches can happen when people feel overwhelmed with too much information, stimulus, and stress. Diffusing the Uranus Planetary Blend or applying a few drops in a clockwise motion can help you find new ways of understanding the world around you and reduce stress when you feel overwhelmed with information. Remember that the tangerine in this blend will increase your sensitivity to sunlight, so use this blend in the evening as the Sun is setting, diffuse it anytime, or apply to the soles of the feet if you are in the sun all day as the skin on the bottom of the feet is thicker and exposed less to the sun.

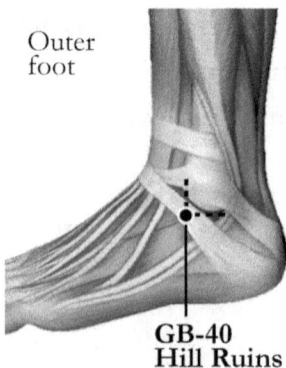

Outer foot

GB-40
Hill Ruins

The acupuncture point Hill Ruins, also known as *Qiu Xu*, Gallbladder 40, or GB-40, is found on the outside of the ankle in the depression just below and anterior to the peak of the outer ankle bone. People with old ankle injuries or who have chronic ankle discomfort may have an area that is swollen and puffy just below the depression. Applying the Uranus Planetary Blend to either of these locations below the ankle in a clockwise motion accesses the energy of Hill Ruins to encourage taking the next steps in life and making needed changes to let your new ideas manifest in physical form. Hill Ruins is the source point for the gallbladder meridian, which means you can add energy into the meridian at this point to help you put your ideas into action. Hill Ruins also activates the entire meridian to harmonize and balance your ability to integrate yourself into your community.

Uranus Planetary Affirmations:

I strive to be an agent of positive change in the world.

I value justice and fairness.

I open my mind to the Divine Mind.

The Neptune Archetype

The Energy of the Planet Neptune and the Liver Meridian

Neptune is the outermost gas giant and the eighth planet from the Sun. It is a beautiful, green-blue planet and has the highest winds of any planet in our solar system. If you listen to the sounds of these winds from the NASA Voyager recordings, they sound like ocean waves.

Archetypally, Neptune is connected with Poseidon (god of the sea), with the waters of the ocean, and with storms. Where Neptune resides in your chart by sign and house is where you may experience "emotional storms." Experiences that dissolve your boundaries may take you into altered states of consciousness. In this way, Neptune is associated with idealism, mysticism, meditation, music, art, and ways in which you can connect with your spirituality and creativity. The shadow side of Neptune is seen in ways that cause you to lose your sense of self or feel emotionally overwhelmed or caught in confusion or in addictions. Whether it is in a conscious or unconscious way, Neptune is where you dissolve your sense of ego and sense of separateness. At its best, it supports you in opening to a profound sense of communion with the oneness of all that is.

Neptune is the ruler of Pisces. In Pisces, Neptune is strongest in manifesting either a deep mysticism, compassion, psychic sensitivity, and idealism or, at its worst, in showing a vulnerability to illusions, escapism, or addictions.

When Neptune is in supportive aspects with other planets, it brings a strong sense of idealism and a desire to be of service. In relationship with the Sun or Moon in particular, Neptune indicates a strong, compassionate, and intuitive nature. Neptune can also manifest in a strong imagination and creativity.

If in more challenging aspects, especially with the Sun or Moon, the Neptunian energy may manifest in feeling emotionally overwhelmed or caught in illusions, having difficulties with boundaries energetically or emotionally, experiencing a vulnerability to addictions or escapism, or experiencing a lack of clear sense of self.

Physically, in modern Western astrology, Neptune is associated with the pineal gland, the third eye, and connections with the spiritual realms. The lymphatic system and feet are also associated with Neptune and the sign of Pisces.

In Chinese medicine, Neptune corresponds with the liver meridian, which controls the flow of *qi* or energy throughout the body, mind, and spirit. When imbalances in this energy system occur, they first manifest as liver *qi* stagnation or blocked energy that affects the emotions and then the physical body. Chinese medicine teaches that emotional imbalances and mental illness occur with physical symptoms and diseases. The liver *qi* moves blood in the body, and the liver organ cleanses the blood. For women, any irregularity or disorder that affects the menstrual cycle disrupts the liver meridian. The meridian system follows along microscopic lymph vessels; the liver *qi* keeps this system balanced and flowing. The liver organ cleanses toxins from the lymph system, thereby supporting the Western association to the lymph system. Environmental toxins, alcohol, prescription medications, processed sugar, and just about anything done to excess negatively impacts the liver meridian.

The Harmonizing Essence of the Neptune Planetary Blend

The planetary blend for Neptune (also known as the Liver Meridian Balancing Blend), consists of 50% bergamot (*Citrus bergamia*), 25% geranium (*Pelargonium graveolens*), and 25% cardamom (*Elettaria cardamomum*). These three essential oils work to harmonize with anything they come into contact with. This can help you to adapt to any situation, strengthen your resolve, and is highly supportive for cleansing toxins, moving stagnant energy, clearing the mind, and releasing negative emotions.

Bergamot is the flavoring used in Earl Grey Tea and is actually part of the citrus family. This citrus targets the third eye and the heart or spirit energy, thereby connecting feelings with psychic abilities. The blood stores your spirit while you sleep, and bergamot supports a restful night's sleep. Bergamot calms the nervous system and is beneficial if you are someone who is highly sensitive, an artist, or someone who struggles with addiction or has a family member who struggles with addiction.

For centuries, people have used geranium to ward off evil spirits, and today it is commonly used to keep away insects and ticks. Geranium adapts to blood viscosity, meaning it "knows" when the blood is too thin or too thick, and the healing properties adjust accordingly to promote the smooth flow of blood throughout the body by supporting the liver *qi*. Geranium cleanses blood to remove xenoestrogens. These are substances that come from plastics; they mimic estrogen in the body and create physical health problems, emotional imbalances, and disruptions in the neurotransmitters of the brain.

Cardamom is a digestive aid that both calms and regenerates the digestive system. Cardamom is a milder plant species in the ginger family and works well for highly sensitive people, pregnant women, and babies. Asian and East Indian cultures use cardamom to calm a nervous stomach and gently support daily detoxification. Cardamom supports the body's removal of problematic xenoestrogens, found throughout the environment. This blend strengthens intuitive and psychic abilities while protecting you from negative influences in your environment that affect the body, mind, and spirit.

How to Use the Neptune Planetary Blend

Many acupuncturists consider the acupuncture point Great Surge, also known as *Tai Chong*, Great Thoroughfare, Large Surge, Liver 3, or LV-3, to be one of the most important acupuncture points. Great Surge is found on the top of the foot, between the first and second toe, in a depression just below the joining of the first and second metatarsal bones, about one or two inches inch proximal (closer to the body) than the webbing of the toes.

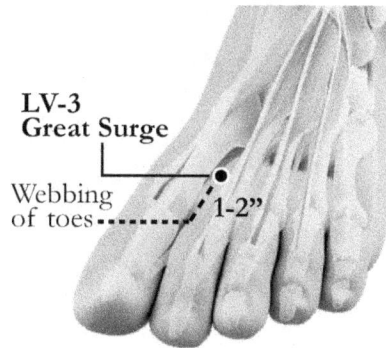

Great Surge pairs with Union Valley, or LI-4, as one of the "Four Gates," to protect the borders of the body. These two points allow energy to both enter and exit the meridian system. Accessing the Four Gates balances and energizes the auric field (the energy field that surrounds your body) and the meridian system. Massaging the Neptune Planetary Blend into the Four Gates point clockwise adds energy to your auric field and calms emotions. Massaging this diluted blend counterclockwise supports releasing toxins and purging negative emotions.

Great Surge is the source point for the liver meridian, which means you can add energy into the meridian at this point to help you strengthen your intuition and creativity. This point is the most commonly used point for hormonal imbalances in the body for both men and women. Applying the Neptune Planetary Blend to Great Surge in an upward and downward motion all the way to the webbing between the first and second toes, will help balance and harmonize all of the meridians and their corresponding emotions.

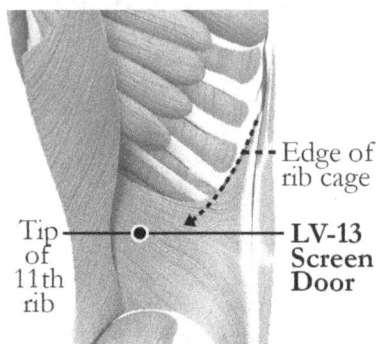

The acupuncture point Screen Door, also known as *Zhang Men*, Camphorwood Gate, Liver 13, or LV-13, is found on the lateral side of the body, at the tip of the eleventh rib. To find this point, follow the lower border of the rib cage around to the side of the body, and your fingers will naturally stop at the tip of the eleventh rib.

Screen Door is the access point to the visceral cavity of the body, which stores your organs. Chinese medicine believes your organs store your subconscious and deep emotions. Screen Door is the influential point and the connecting point of the internal organs and the alarm point of the spleen and pancreas organs. Screen Door connects the liver and gallbladder meridians and is an access point for the *Dai Mai* or Girdling Vessel. One of the eight extra vessels, *Dai Mai* harmonizes the upper half of the body (where the spirit dwells) with the lower half (where we live in the physical world).

Applying this blend in a two or three-inch diameter to Screen Door will harmonize your internal organs and the deep thought patterns found in your subconscious. This blend can help you identify and transform negative or limiting internal dialogue that relates to challenging Neptune aspects. When used with beneficial Neptune aspects, this blend energizes your creativity and intuition.

Since bergamot is part of the citrus family, it will increase the effects of the sun where applied during the day. Applying the Neptune Planetary Blend to the soles of the feet, which are usually not exposed to sunlight, at any time of the day will help you ground your soul to this Earthly world in a safe way.

Neptune Planetary Affirmations:	I open to oneness with all of Life and to Spirit. I allow love to flow through me. I am sensitive to others but clear with my own boundaries.

The Pluto Archetype

The Energy of the Planet Pluto and the Kidney Meridian

Pluto is the smallest planet in our solar system and has recently been demoted to the status of a dwarf planet, yet, archetypally, its meaning and power are undiminished. Pluto is a rocky planet and is one-third water in the form of ice.

Pluto is the modern ruler of the sign Scorpio. In ancient mythology, the constellation of Scorpio (or Scorpius) represents the threshold between life and death. These stars lie near the black rift in the Milky Way, our connection to the Galactic Center. The center of our galaxy is a black hole from which all life in our galaxy was born. It carries the energy of creation and destruction, birthing all that is and taking everything back into itself in a cycle of life/death/rebirth. When Pluto is in Scorpio, it shows depth, intensity, and commitment to being in an ongoing process of transformation.

Pluto is associated with the god of the underworld, and where Pluto resides in your chart by house and sign is where you are called to dive deep and to be open to transformation. Pluto, in evolutionary astrology, is the planet that shows you where you have been striving to grow and evolve spiritually. Pluto teaches you how not to be afraid of the intense and transformational experiences in your life and shows you how to move through the cycle of life/death/rebirth in all its forms. Pluto represents the energy of alchemy and the transmutation of lead to gold and helps you to find the true gold, the unique essence, of who you are. As the caterpillar needs to dissolve in order to be reborn as the butterfly, so it is important to release patterns and ways of being that no longer serve you in order to open to the transformation and deepening of consciousness that Pluto offers.

When you work with Pluto consciously and have beneficial aspects to this planet (especially with the Sun or Moon) and allow its energy to support you, it may guide you in having a profound capacity to heal and regenerate even after a life-threatening illness or crisis. Pluto will support you in living from your true essence and deeper purpose and in "burning off" patterns and ways of being that no longer serve you.

If you resist Pluto's energy or are caught in challenging aspects with this planet, it is possible to get mired in turmoil and toxic emotional experiences. Archetypally, Pluto is the planet that represents power. At its best, it is supporting you in becoming empowered and in living from your deeper soul self. If it is out of balance, Pluto can lead to becoming embroiled in power struggles, abusive dynamics, or acting in self-destructive ways.

Physically, Pluto governs the regenerative energy of physical and psychological healing. It is associated with catabolism and anabolism or the death and rebirth of cells in the body. It supports you in releasing toxins and in growing a new body every seven years. Diseases associated with Pluto relate to autoimmune disorders or toxicity in the body.

In Chinese medicine, Pluto corresponds to the kidney meridian, which, of all the meridians, influences the aging process the most. Cellular aging reflects the life force inside your cells and denotes overall health and longevity. The kidney meridian influences the endocrine system and the adrenal glands, which sit atop the kidneys. How you handle stress directly impacts the adrenal glands and cellular aging. The kidney meridian also influences reproduction, the teeth, and the bones. All of which are seen as indicators of cellular aging at different stages of life. Western medicine now calculates cellular aging by measuring the ends of DNA strands called telomeres.

The kidney meridian pairs with the heart meridian to regulate the deepest levels of the body, those that house your spirit and your life force, known as deepest yin. Many of the kidney meridian points affect your emotional health, spirit, and life force. Supporting the kidney and heart meridians will help you process major changes in your life. The greatest sources of stress are transformational times in life, such as the birth of a child, the death of a parent or family member, career changes, or moving. A balanced kidney meridian supports a healthy stress response during times of transition and transformation. It also slows the cellular aging process and aligns you to natural rhythms of graceful aging.

The Harmonizing Essence of the Pluto Planetary Blend

The Pluto Planetary Blend (also known as the Kidney Meridian Balancing Blend) consists of 50% cedarwood (*Cedrus atlantica*), 25% sandalwood (*Santalum album*), and 25% carrot seed (*Daucus carota*). These three essential oils contain the highest levels of sesquiterpene alcohols, offering the highest capacity for regeneration of the endocrine system, brain, and internal organs. This blend targets the endocrine glands in the brain, including the hypothalamus, pineal, and pituitary glands, which influence how you perceive the world around you. All three of these oils harmonize and balance the different hemispheres of the brain to encourage healthy communication of the nervous system. All three are beneficial for the skin and diluting them with a carrier oil, or non-toxic lotion creates a regenerative moisturizer with a beautiful aroma.

Cedarwood regulates the cortisol and melatonin cycles, which control energy production and focus during the day and the ability to rest and sleep at night. Cedarwood supports a healthy response to stress by soothing the amygdala's fight or flight response and activating the frontal lobe for logical processing. A good night's sleep, the ability to concentrate, and an appropriate stress response are critical to handling Pluto's transformational energies. Cedarwood encourages the proper balance of male and female hormones and is beneficial for any hormonal imbalance affecting the skin.

Churches and spiritual groups around the world use sandalwood for sacred ceremonies, funerals, and meditation. Perfumers use sandalwood essential oil for its alluring aroma. In Chinese medicine, sandalwood adds to your life force and promotes feelings of safety and security.

Essential oils contain the highest life force of a plant; the second highest life force is found in the seeds of a plant. One of the best ways to support your life force is by sprouting the seeds of plants to activate their life force then eating them. Carrot seed supports healthy eyesight, and when combined with cedarwood can help you see things from a different perspective. Carrot seed encourages new insights during times of change; it cools the blood vessels and capillaries that feed the skin and eyes for a cool-headed approach to Pluto's challenges.

How to Use the Pluto Planetary Blend

Three consecutive points found together on the kidney meridian house the spirit inside the body. The three points are Spirit Seal, Spirit Ruins, and Spirit Storehouse. Collectively, they contain, nourish, and transform energy to store your spirit. The first point, Spirit Seal, houses the yang or masculine aspects of your spirit and creates the container that houses and protects your spirit. The second point, Spirit Ruins, provides nourishment for and houses the yin or feminine aspects of your spirit. The third point, Spirit Storehouse, holds your integrated spirit, which comes from harmonizing Spirit Seal and Spirit Ruins along with the spirit energy of each of the internal organs.

These points are found on the chest, about two inches from the midline of the body, just lateral to where the rib cage meets the

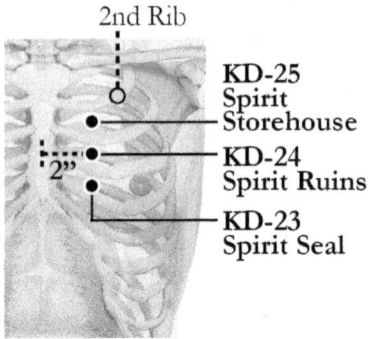

2nd Rib

KD-25
Spirit
Storehouse

KD-24
Spirit Ruins

KD-23
Spirit Seal

2"

sternum. The acupuncture point Spirit Seal, also known as *Shen Feng*, Kidney 23, or KD-23, is found below the fourth rib; on men, this point sits at the same level as the nipple. Spirit Ruins, also known as *Ling Xi*, Spirit Wall, Kidney 24, or KD-24, is found below the third rib. Spirit Storehouse, also known as *Shen Cang*, Kidney 25, or KD-25, is found below the second rib.

Spirit Seal, Spirit Ruins, and Spirit Storehouse become tender with high levels of stress, with congested lymph nodes, and when the cardiovascular system needs support. Applying a few drops of the Pluto Planetary Blend, diluted with either a non-toxic lotion or carrier oil, in a clockwise circle that encompasses these three points and the breastbone creates a protective and nurturing barrier for your spirit. This blend diluted with non-toxic lotions or carrier oils creates a nice rejuvenating moisturizer for the face, neck, and chest. Diffusing this blend at night is a perfect option for children and for accessing the transformational power of the subconscious.

Pluto Planetary Affirmations:

I align my will with Divine Will.

I am open to diving deep and transforming.

I allow my life experiences to deepen my spiritual growth.

The Chiron Archetype

The Energy of Chiron and the Small Intestine Meridian

Chiron moves between the orbits of Saturn and Uranus. Formerly known as an asteroid, it is now known as a minor planet in a new class of objects called "centaurs" (minor planets orbiting between the asteroid belt and the Kuiper belt). Since it exhibits behavior similar to a comet, Chiron is also classified as a comet.

In Greek mythology, Chiron was a centaur (half human and half horse) who was a wise teacher and healer. He was accidentally wounded in the heel with a deadly arrow shot by Hercules. He was immortal, so he did not die but lived on in chronic pain. He was finally freed from his pain after trading his life to save Prometheus. Chiron is therefore symbolic of the wounded healer.

Where Chiron resides in your chart (by house, sign, and aspects) reflects a core emotional wound, either from early in this lifetime or a karmic wound. When you face this wound and work through the healing process, Chiron also represents your healing gifts.

In beneficial aspects with other planets, Chiron's influence helps you to heal those areas of life and to manifest your healing gifts. For example, Chiron in close aspect to the Sun may indicate that you are someone who experienced early wounds that affected your sense of self but perhaps you have grown up to become a healer.

In more challenging aspects with other planets, Chiron again shows areas where you may experience emotional wounds or carry karmic wounds from the past. It helps you to heal these issues in order to grow and evolve and then share that compassion and healing energy with others.

In Western astrology, Chiron is different than the planets in the birth chart and is not associated with any particular physical part of the body, but rather shows where the person may experience early or karmic core emotional wounds.

In Chinese medicine, Chiron corresponds with the small intestine meridian, which pairs with the heart meridian that stores the spirit. When the small intestine meridian is out of balance, the heart meridian is negatively affected, and the spirit becomes irritated or restless. The small intestine meridian influences the digestive system, the endocrine system, and brain function. The relationship between digestive health and mental health occurs through the small intestine meridian. In the digestive system, the small intestine meridian is responsible for the first stages of separating nutrients from food and assimilating most of them. The corresponding emotional function separates the beneficial opportunities or lessons from the negative ones to support continued emotional growth for the spirit.

The Harmonizing Essence of the Chiron Planetary Blend

The Chiron Planetary Blend (also known as the Small Intestine Meridian Balancing Blend) consists of 50% ylang ylang (*Cananga odorata*), 25% vetiver (*Vetiveria zizanoides*), and 25% copaiba (copal: *Copaifera reticulate* or *Copaifera L. genus*). All three of these oils are beneficial for the skin and for scars of any type. In Chinese medicine, scars hold the memory of both emotional and physical trauma. Scars that are painful can cause blockages in the meridian system and disrupt the flow of *qi* or energy throughout the body. Trauma to the body causes both a scar or irritation on the skin's surface and a corresponding deeper scar in the muscle, connective tissue, or bone. The skin can easily shift during trauma and surgeries, causing an internal scar at a slightly different area from the external scar. Be sure to check both the scar on the skin and the area around it to find deeper scarring.

Vetiver assists in releasing cellular memories of traumatic stress and physical trauma. Because vetiver works on a cellular level, it can also release unconscious stored memories to encourage emotional growth. Vetiver is a type of grass that supports your healthy bacterial flora in the small intestine, needed for digestion. Ylang ylang and copaiba transform vetiver's intense aroma to a softer appealing aroma that you can wear as perfume.

Copaiba calms irritation in the body and supports the normal healing process that follows an injury. Copaiba relieves stress and nervous tension; it calms the mind to allow for clear thinking to process emotions in a healthy way. Copaiba strengthens the Chiron Planetary Blend by enhancing the effects of the other oils, thereby increasing the strength of this blend.

You can use the Chiron Planetary Blend at any time. The stimulating properties of copaiba balance the sedating properties of vetiver. Vetiver and copaiba target the deeper layers of the body to release trauma, stored memories, and adhesions caused by scarring.

In Chinese medicine, ylang ylang balances the male and female energies along with optimizing hormonal balance and regulating mood swings. Ylang ylang is one of the strongest harmonizing essential oils, and used in this blend, it adapts to release any old trauma affecting the body and spirit. All three of these oils revitalize the skin for scars, aging, acne, and irritation.

How to Use the Chiron Planetary Blend

Diffusing or wearing the Chiron Planetary Blend during either the day or the night will calm the mind to promote focus or a restful night's sleep. Diluting this blend with a non-toxic lotion or carrier oil is ideal for the skin. Apply it over any scars to release the cellular memories of the trauma. Add a few drops of this blend to a non-toxic facial moisturizer for rejuvenation and clear thinking.

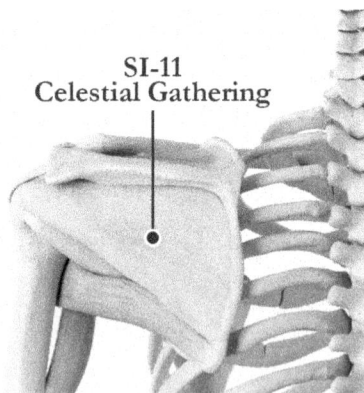

SI-11
Celestial Gathering

Two acupuncture points on the small intestine meridian, Celestial Gathering and Celestial Window, support the connection to your spirit or higher self and help process physical and emotional trauma. Celestial Gathering, also known as *Tian Zong*, Small Intestine 11, or SI-11, is found on the upper back over the center of both scapula bones. This point over the left scapula connects to the heart and stores your spirit. The Celestial Gathering point becomes congested with physical and emotional trauma and stores cellular memories. Accessing this point helps you to take control of emotional situations. Applying the Chiron Planetary Blend in a clockwise circle over the left scapula will help you process through stored traumatic memories held at the Celestial Gathering point.

The acupuncture point Celestial Window, also known as *Tian Rong*, Small Intestine 16, or SI-16, is found on the neck behind the sternocleidomastoid muscle on the same level as the Adam's Apple (laryngeal prominence). Celestial Window is a window of Heaven point, which provides access to the spirit or higher self to treat emotional imbalances. Wearing the Chiron Planetary Blend here as perfume calms the spirit and supports the processing of emotional stress. The Celestial Window point is close to the ear and promotes clarity in hearing the deeper meaning of messages in conversations. If you are a healer or have aspects to Chiron in your birth chart, accessing Celestial Window with the Chiron Planetary Blend can help you to help others process their emotional wounds.

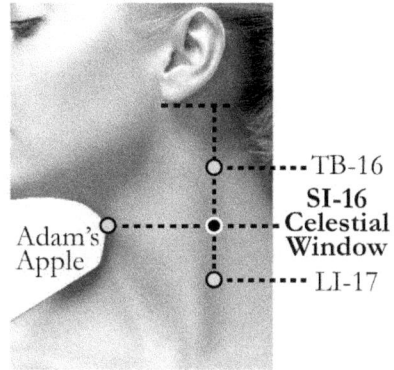

Chiron Planetary Affirmations:	I am open to working on my core wounds.
	I accept my vulnerabilities and am compassionate with others.
	I honor my healing gifts.

Archetypes of the Signs of the Zodiac

We will now introduce you to the archetypal meanings of the signs of the zodiac. Find your sun and moon signs below to deepen your understanding of the energies of your identity and emotional nature. Also, you may want to look at the other planets in your chart and integrate the meaning of each planet (or that facet of yourself) with the meaning of the sign that it is in. Use the sign essential oil blends in combination with your Sun and Moon planetary blends to support your core essence and to be in balance emotionally and physically. Or use the sign oil blend to strengthen the energy of a planet that is in that sign or to help you with physical or emotional imbalances related to the organ associated with that sign.

The following table shows the time of the year for each sign of the zodiac, its element, modality, and core archetypal meaning:

Sign	Approximate Dates	Element	Modality	Archetypal Meaning
ARIES	Mar 21–Apr 20	Fire	Cardinal	Action Initiative
TAURUS	Apr 21–May 20	Earth	Fixed	Embodiment
GEMINI	May 21–Jun 20	Air	Mutable	Communication
CANCER	Jun 21–Jul 21	Water	Cardinal	Feeling Nurturing
LEO	Jul 22–Aug 22	Fire	Fixed	Creativity Self-expression
VIRGO	Aug 23–Sep 22	Earth	Mutable	Discernment Service
LIBRA	Sep 23–Oct 22	Air	Cardinal	Relationship Balance
SCORPIO	Oct 23–Nov 21	Water	Fixed	Transformation
SAGITTARIUS	Nov 22–Dec 20	Fire	Mutable	Exploration Beliefs
CAPRICORN	Dec 21–Jan 20	Earth	Cardinal	Accomplishment
AQUARIUS	Jan 21–Feb 18	Air	Fixed	Social reform Innovation
PISCES	Feb 19–Mar 20	Water	Mutable	Compassion Spirituality Intuition

The Birth Chart: Angles and Their Signs

The Ascendant and Descendant constitute the horizontal axis in the birth chart and indicate the horizon line at the time of birth. The Midheaven or Medium Coeli (MC) and the Root of the chart or Imum Coeli (IC) form the vertical axis. These axes mark the four directions and are central factors in the chart. The Ascendant and Descendant form the East/West axis while the MC and IC show the South/North axis.

Below is Allie's birth chart showing the location of the horizontal and vertical axes in her chart:

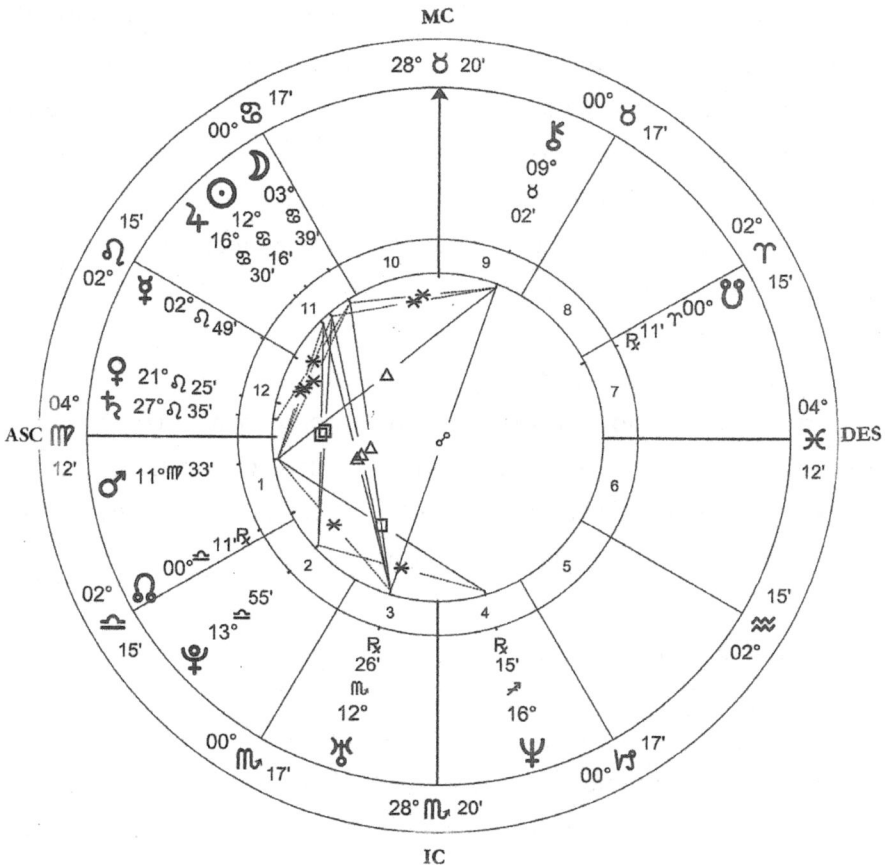

Allie's Birth Chart

To find the signs of the zodiac on the angles of your chart, first identify the horizontal axis then look at the sign to the left of this line in the outer wheel. This is your Ascendant. Then, look at the sign on the right in the outer wheel for the sign of the Descendant. Looking at the vertical dark line through the middle of the chart, the sign on the top is the midheaven, and the sign at the bottom of that line is the IC (Imum Coeli).

ASCENDANT (ASC)

The Ascendant in the birth chart is associated with the direction of the East and the time of sunrise. The sign on your Ascendant indicates the energies and influences at the time of your birth as well as the persona or way in which you present yourself to the world and how you interact with others. If planets are in conjunction with the Ascendant, they represent core aspects of who you are. From a physical perspective, the sign on the Ascendant and its planetary ruler (and its aspects in the chart) indicate your vitality and general health.

You may want to use the sign oil blend associated with your Ascendant to support you in how you interact with others and to improve your physical and emotional health. If you have planets close to the Ascendant, use that planetary blend in conjunction with the sign blend of the Ascendant.

DESCENDANT (DES)

The Descendant marks the direction of the West and the time of sunset. It reflects what you seek in relationship with others and may indicate the archetypal energy of your primary relationship or partner (or your ideal for a partner). Often, planets on the

Descendant show aspects of yourself that you may tend to project onto others. It is important to become conscious of these qualities being core aspects of who you are.

MIDHEAVEN (MC)

The Midheaven marks the highest point in the chart and is associated with the direction of the South and the time of noon. The sign of the Midheaven gives information about how you bring your gifts out into the world and how you shine in a visible way. It also indicates the type of career that you might be drawn to and how you present yourself in the world.

If you want to support your work in the world and to live out your gifts at the highest potential, use the sign oil blend that is associated with the sign of your Midheaven. If you have a planet next to the Midheaven, combine that planetary blend with the sign oil blend for your Midheaven.

ROOT OF THE CHART (IC)

The Imum Coeli is associated with the direction of the North and the time of midnight. It indicates what your roots are in terms of your ancestral lineage as well as the themes in your family of origin. This part of the chart is also connected with what you need to feel grounded in the world (including your sense of home) and the foundation of your sense of self.

If you are working through emotional issues related to your early childhood and family environment, karmic issues related to your ancestral lineage or health problems stemming from your genetic inheritance, use the sign oil blend associated with the IC in your chart to support you in your healing process.

The Signs of the Zodiac and Their Meaning

Following are the descriptions of the signs of the zodiac and their core archetypal energies. Use this section to deepen your understanding of your sun sign and moon sign as well as the energies of the signs that your planets are in.

The Aries Archetype

The Energy of the Sign of Aries and the Lung Organ

Aries, the Ram, is a cardinal fire sign. Here in the northern hemisphere, it carries the energy of the beginning of spring when the heat in the Earth is bursting forth in new life after the long months of winter. Aries embodies the energy of new beginnings and of taking action. Aries will seize the moment by taking the initiative and by jumping into situations, often without thinking through the consequences first. Aries represents the fire of new birth, of inspiration, and the excitement of exploration and adventure.

If you have strong Aries energy in your birth chart and are living with self-awareness and at a higher vibrational level, you are likely to have strong leadership skills, and you may be a pioneer or trailblazer. In balance with Aries energy, you are apt to be assertive and comfortable taking risks. You may be self-confident and comfortable initiating projects. You are likely to have a strong will and are quick to take action.

If out of balance or if you have strong Aries energy in your chart and are operating with less consciousness, you may tend to be impulsive or reactive. You may jump into situations without thinking through the consequences and then find yourself in "hot water." You may also be quick to anger, but the feelings are likely to pass quickly as you move on to new experiences. You may have trouble being sensitive to others' feelings and needs and tend to be strong-willed and self-focused.

From an astrological perspective, each sign is balanced by the one opposite it in the astrological chart. For Aries, the balancing sign is Libra, guiding you to integrate the two signs, to be aware of the needs and feelings of others, and not to be overly focused on yourself. With the energies of Aries and Libra in balance, you have the ability to assert yourself while valuing balance and harmony in your relationships.

The ruler of Aries is Mars and this planet functions in a strong and clear way when in this sign. Mars in Aries indicates decisiveness and an ability to take action in effective ways.

In Western astrology, Aries is physically associated with the head and, under stress, may manifest in headaches.

In Chinese medicine, Aries corresponds to the lung organ. The lungs are sensitive and tender and open to the world to give energy form, structure, and definition. When the lungs are strong the spirit feels inspired, the skin is vibrant, and the body has abundant power, even tempo, and superior immunity. Under stress, the lungs can cause feelings of grief, an inappropriate sense of boundaries, and scattered energies. If your Aries Sun, Moon, or Ascendant has challenging aspects, you may experience constitutional or genetic issues affecting the lungs such as pneumonia, allergies, asthma, or other respiratory problems.

Key Themes for Aries Sun, Moon, and Ascendant

ARIES SUN:

The Sun relates to our essential identity. When the sun is in Aries, your core sense of self and constitution reflect the energy of this cardinal fire sign.

When worked consciously and in balance, your Aries Sun can manifest as your being able to be independent and confident, with leadership abilities and the capacity to take action in an effective way in the world. Many leaders, pioneers, innovators, or those who are willing to take risks for new enterprises, have strong Aries energy. When your sun sign is Aries, you are likely to have a strong will and your actions are consistent with who you are. You are direct and forthright and enjoy physical activity.

If the Aries Sun is challenged through transits or other planetary aspects, you may have difficulties with self-confidence and self-assertion. You may also have unresolved grief and low self-esteem. Or, under stress, your Aries Sun may manifest as being overly focused on your own needs and insensitive to others.

Stressful aspects or transits may also increase the "headstrong" qualities of Aries such as your insistence on doing things your own way or your tendency to get into conflict easily. Often, these underlying issues around a lack of self-esteem or an insecure sense of self, stemming from a challenging relationship with your father in childhood and a lack of feeling valued or affirmed in that relationship.

ARIES MOON:

The Moon relates to our ways of experiencing and expressing our emotions as well as our physical and emotional health. When the Moon is in Aries, your emotional functioning and health issues are influenced by the Aries energy. Often your feelings will be fiery or manifest in your actions. Your moods can shift rapidly and are related to what is happening in the moment. You may enjoy physical activity and need to exercise to reduce stress. You may also find it helpful to express your feelings or release stress through movement such as dance, walking meditation, or running.

If worked consciously, the Aries Moon can give you emotional strength, independence, and a high level of energy. You tend to have a positive attitude about life and feel upbeat. Emotions tend to surface rapidly and pass quickly, and you are not likely to brood or hang on to emotions or resentments. You may tend to be quick to anger, but then the frustration or anger is likely to dissipate rapidly. You are comfortable with conflict or confrontation and tend to be direct and assertive in how you interact with others. You like physical activity and find this a good outlet for reducing stress.

With challenging aspects to your Aries Moon, you may have difficulty being aware of your emotions and be quick to anger. For some with a challenging Aries Moon, anger covers underlying feelings of grief or low self-esteem. You may feel depressed or have low energy. Or you may have experienced your mother as moody and not supportive of you emotionally, resulting in feelings of insecurity and difficulties with asserting yourself. Out of balance or not working with this aspect consciously, you may also be insensitive to others' feelings and needs and tend to be impatient, reactive, and prone to conflict. You may experience headaches or feel like your energy is blocked. Physical activity and exercise are good ways to channel and release emotions and reduce stress.

ARIES ASCENDANT:
The Ascendant is the third foundation point of the birth chart and relates to another facet of identity, including your birth experience, vitality, and how you engage with others.

When in balance, the Aries Ascendant may manifest in your being active, wiry, independent, and assertive in how you come across and interact with others. There is a natural tendency to take the initiative, to be willing to take risks, and to move into positions of leadership.

When in challenging aspects, transits, or under stress with the Aries Ascendant, you may have difficulties with taking risks or asserting yourself. In interacting with others, you may also tend to be either overly assertive (or angry and aggressive) or to have difficulty taking action or being direct with your feelings and needs.

In Western astrology, when under stress the Aries Ascendant may manifest lung issues, respiratory problems, headaches, or migraines.

The Harmonizing Essence of the Aries Sign Blend

The Aries Sign Blend (also known as the Lung Organ Supporting Blend) consists of 40% lemon (*Citrus limon*), 40% lemon myrtle

(*Backhousia citriodora*), 10% basil (*Ocimum basilicum*), and 10% peppermint (*Mentha piperita*). The synergistic effects of the Aries Sign Blend promote clear direction and forward movement while harmonizing with others to support the independent and free-spirited nature of those who are born with an Aries Sun, Moon, or Ascendant. The cleansing properties of these four oils are perfect for enhancing a spring detoxifying cleanse and for diffusing while spring cleaning. Inhaling this blend will boost your cortisol and get you moving, making it a perfect way to start your day or enhance your exercise routine.

Peppermint and basil oils are high in phenols, which cleanse and activate the cellular receptor sites to allow nutrients and hormones to enter the cells. Aries often craves cleansing on an emotional and physical level, and this blend triggers cleansing by starting with the individual cells. In Chinese medicine, peppermint and basil are exterior releasing, which boosts a healthy immune response to protect the borders of the body and cool the skin. This supports Aries's love for the outdoors and physical activities.

Basil essential oil releases tension from the head, neck, and shoulders, common areas for your Aries Sun, Moon, or Ascendant to hold stress. This oil has unique properties that allow it to stimulate the mind and relax the muscles simultaneously. Basil supports healthy lung function to encourage full and deep breathing.

Lemon essential oil is emotionally uplifting and clarifying for the mind to give your Aries Sun, Moon, or Ascendant clear vision and direction for the future. Both lemon and lemon myrtle essential oils clear excessive mucus, phlegm, congestion, and stagnant fluids from the sinuses, head, lungs, and reproductive organs. Together these oils enhance the positive attributes of your Aries Sun, Moon, or Ascendant and help you to harmonize with the rest of the zodiac.

How to Use the Aries Sign Blend

The Aries Sign Blend is high in phenols and contains a citrus oil, both of which can irritate the skin but are perfect for cleansing the air. Basil, lemon, and peppermint are stimulating both physically and mentally. Therefore, diffusing this blend upon waking and anytime you're looking for a pick-me-up is ideal. Applying the Aries Sign Blend to the soles of the feet can help you take those first steps in the morning with added energy, or help when you are looking for a new direction in life.

In Chinese medicine, the corporeal soul, called *po*, embodies the non-physical aspect of every living being and enables the body to move and feel physical sensations. The corporeal soul allows you to express animation and drives instinctual behaviors. The lung organ stores the corporeal soul and permits newborns to begin breathing and take in milk. The acupuncture alarm point for the lung organ is Central Treasury, also known as Center Storehouse, which means this is the storage place of *po* energy for the body.

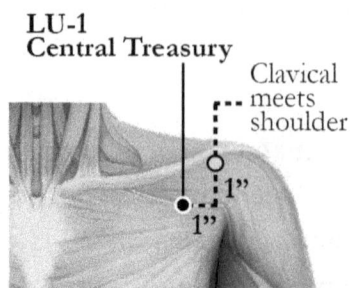

LU-1
Central Treasury
Clavical meets shoulder
1"
1"

The acupuncture point Central Treasury, also known as *Zhong Fu*, Lung 1, or LU-1, is found on the lateral side of the chest about one inch below and one inch towards the center of the body from where the clavicle bone meets the shoulder joint. This point becomes tender when the corporeal soul or lung organ is out of balance with the environment or the other meridians, and it acts as an alarm point for issues affecting the skin.

Tenderness at the Central Treasury acupuncture point indicates different things for people with a strong Aries influence. For the Aries Sun, this tenderness may indicate low physical energy and lack of reserves to work towards their goals. For the Aries Moon, this tenderness may indicate feeling emotionally spent or easily disappointed or offended. For the Aries Ascendant, this tenderness may indicate struggles with respiratory issues or taking the initiative.

Diffusing or applying the Aries Sign Blend to the soles of the feet can help relieve tension stored at Central Treasury and allow the corporeal soul freedom of expression. Diluting this blend with a carrier oil and applying it directly over Central Treasury in a clockwise motion helps to harmonize home, family, and work life. Working with the Aries Sign Blend affirmations brings intention and an improved sense of self when spoken out loud and into the mirror.

| *The Aries Sign Blend Affirmations:* | I honor who I am and my uniqueness.

I am inspired to live life to the fullest.

I take action in a careful way. |

The Taurus Archetype

The Energy of the Sign of Taurus and the Large Intestine Organ

Taurus, the Bull, is a fixed earth sign and comes as spring moves into its fullness. This is the time when the Earth manifests her beauty in the flowers and budding trees. Taurus represents your sense of self-worth and your ability to feel comfortable in your own skin and in tune with who you are physically. It also relates to your external resources as well as your internal values. The energy of Taurus is about being able to enjoy the beauty of life and the joys of embodiment.

If in balance, the energy of Taurus indicates that you are likely to be a person who is grounded, practical, and reliable. The fixed nature of this sign brings a sense of stability and the capacity to persevere in order to manifest what is important in life. If you have a Taurus sun sign, you may feel nurtured through your connection with nature and by being in a comfortable and beautiful home environment. Taurus is also associated with the arts, such as pottery and cooking, that involve a sensual, tangible experience of creativity.

If out of balance, Taurus energy can manifest in feeling stuck, having difficulty making changes, or being overly focused on finances or material resources for a sense of security. Being uncomfortable physically or with body image as well as having low self-esteem are other manifestations of being out of balance with Taurus energy.

The ruler of Taurus is Venus and is associated with our relationships with self and others. The sign opposite Taurus is Scorpio, which helps us to manifest our lives with depth and more emotional awareness. In balancing Taurus with Scorpio, we are encouraged to realize that everything in our lives has its "season," and that life is a process of moving through change, of endings and new beginnings.

In Western astrology, Taurus is physically associated with the throat, so imbalances or stresses may relate to throat or thyroid issues or with difficulties expressing your truth or "voice."

In Chinese medicine, Taurus corresponds to the large intestine organ, also referred to as the colon. The final stages of digestion occur in the large intestine, where your healthy bacterial flora absorb B-Vitamins and other nutrients. Then fiber, waste, toxins, and used hormone metabolites are released. When the large intestine is healthy, the body and spirit extract all that is beneficial from life's experiences and let go of situations that are no longer useful. As seen with other digestive organs, both emotional stress and poor-quality foods can challenge the large intestine and contribute to constipation or loose stools. If your Taurus Sun, Moon, or Ascendant has challenging aspects, you may find yourself holding on to people, places, or things that are not beneficial to you, or letting go of those that are beneficial too quickly. Physically you may struggle with irregular bowel movements and lower back pain in the morning.

Key Themes for Taurus Sun, Moon, and Ascendant

TAURUS SUN:

If your Sun is in Taurus and you are working this energy in a conscious way, you are likely to have a stable sense of yourself and strong values that you live by. You are apt to be grounded, dependable, and practical. You are someone others rely on to get things done, and you are adept at manifesting your goals. You may value having a stable home base and having a sense of financial and physical security.

If your Taurus Sun is out of balance or in challenging aspects, Sun in Taurus may manifest as a fear of change and a tendency to be stubborn and a reluctance to take risks. You may be too tied to finances and physical resources for your sense of security, and lack a deeper sense of the meaning of life or of your purpose.

TAURUS MOON:

If your Moon is in Taurus and in balance, you are likely to be emotionally stable. You tend to be calm and even-tempered. You are not easily unsettled by stress or by others' emotions since you tend to be emotionally secure and grounded. You are likely to enjoy being surrounded by colors, comfortable furniture, and beautiful objects. You love touch and value sensuality and the joy of experiencing life through the senses. You may feel nurtured by spending time in nature or eating a delicious meal.

If your Taurus Moon is out of balance or not worked consciously, you may have difficulty being aware of your emotions at a deeper level. You may also tend to be inflexible and to want things to be consistent in your life in order to feel secure. You may see your self-worth as linked with your finances and physical resources. You may collect things and have difficulty releasing objects in your life that no longer serve you. If upset, you may hang on to feelings of distress and have difficulty letting go.

Also, if your Taurus Moon is in challenging aspects or transits, you may experience stress through body symptoms and become overly focused on your physical sensations, while lacking a deeper understanding of the mind-body connection.

TAURUS ASCENDANT:

If your Taurus Ascendant is in balance, you are grounded and stable in your interactions with others. Others view you as reliable and trustworthy. You tend not to be moody or inconsistent, and you live guided by your strong values and ethics. You are likely to be self-confident with a strong sense of your gifts and abilities. You are resilient and resourceful.

If your Taurus Ascendant is out of balance or not lived consciously, the Taurus Ascendant can manifest in being strong-willed and stubborn, demanding to have your own way in order to feel secure. It may also manifest in being overly focused on financial success without thinking through the deeper purpose of your gifts. You may also be fearful of change and uncomfortable with changes in your daily routine. You may tend to hang on to feelings or objects with a fear of letting go or fear of feeling deprived or because of underlying feelings of inadequacy or insecurity.

Physically, if in balance, the Taurus Ascendant manifests in good health, and you are able to withstand stress physically and emotionally more easily than others.

The Harmonizing Essence of the Taurus Sign Blend

The Taurus Sign Blend (also known as the Large Intestine Organ Supporting Blend) consists of 40% jade lemon (*Citrus limon eureka var. formosensis*), 40% hinoki (*Chamaecyparis obtusa*), 10% lemon myrtle (*Backhousia citriodora*), and 10% spearmint (*Mentha spicata*). If needed, you can substitute lemon (*Citrus limon*) for jade lemon and cypress (*Cupressus sempervirens*) for hinoki. These four oils together instill a cleansing floral sweetness that resonates so purely with Taurus that they feel right at home when smelling and wearing this blend. This blend fosters the needed changes this fixed earth sign often struggles to make, by energetically moving and grounding simultaneously. Uplifting the emotions with the jade lemon and lemon myrtle, while also promoting circulation and grounding with the hinoki and spearmint, this blend makes it easier for the Taurus Sun, Moon, or Ascendant to let go and move past challenges that have held them back.

The aroma from the exotic plant species of jade lemon, hinoki, and lemon myrtle are richer than their everyday counterpart oils (lemon, cypress, and myrtle), which suit the Taurus Sun, Moon, or Ascendant's appreciation of the finer things in life.

Jade lemon and hinoki (or lemon and cypress) essential oils support healthy detoxification by relieving congestion, excessive fluid accumulation, and mucus, which can easily build up from eating a rich or excessively sweet diet that Taurus is naturally drawn to. Spearmint can also curb cravings as it boosts metabolism to support a healthy weight and body image. If your brand of oils is approved for internal use, then adding a few drops of lemon and spearmint to water with meals can support healthy digestion and assimilation of nutrients.

In Chinese medicine, the sign of Taurus corresponds with the colon, sinuses, and the immune system. The releasing properties of the lemon myrtle and the cypress help the colon to release what is no longer needed. Spearmint stimulates cortisol and energy production to encourage both physical and mental activity making it the perfect morning blend. All four of these oils support a healthy and balanced immune system while opening up the sinuses. Diffusing the Taurus Sign Blend at the first sign of congestion and feeling stagnant will help you to get moving.

How to Use the Taurus Sign Blend

Diffusing the exotic oils of the Taurus Sign Blend lifts your Taurus's Sun, Moon, or Ascendant spirits while promoting feelings of gratitude. The ideal time to use this blend is in the morning to energize and motivate the fixed nature of this sign. Applying this blend over the lower back supports healthy elimination, and applying it to the soles of the feet supports moving forward and increased metabolism. Start the day on the right foot by setting your intentions for the day while applying or diffusing this blend.

Cautions: the Taurus Sign Blend includes lemon essential oil (a citrus) and so may increase photosensitivity in the applied area. You will need to diffuse this blend or apply it to an area that doesn't receive direct exposure to sunlight if you live in a sunny climate, are going to expose the application site to the sun, or have sun-damaged skin. If you have sensitive skin, remember to dilute this blend 50/50 with a carrier oil when applying to the lower abdomen or lower back.

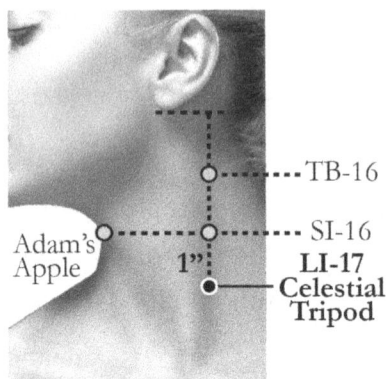

The acupuncture point Celestial Tripod, also known as *Tian Ding*, Large Intestine 17, and LI-17, is found on the side of the neck behind the sternocleidomastoid muscle about one inch below the level of the Adam's Apple. Apply oil to an alternative site if you have sun damaged skin on your neck or will be in the sun. The Chinese character for *Ding* describes an Ancient Chinese sacred cooking vessel with two ear-like extensions for handles that was supported by three legs. This exquisite vessel housed the brain, "the storehouse of the original spirit," atop a three-legged stand.[6] The character *Tian* represents the heavens, celestial influences, and nature.[7] Celestial Tripod personifies Taurus's appreciation for the finer things in life, such as the arts and fine dining, while remaining stable and balanced on the sacred trinity of the father, son, and holy ghost, or the maiden, mother, and crone.

In Chinese medicine, Celestial Tripod treats disorders of the neck, loss of voice, sore throat, and thyroid disorders. If you have a strong Taurus influence in your chart, you may find yourself clearing your throat from either post-nasal drip, sinus congestion, or emotionally feeling held back from speaking your truth. Apply the Taurus Sign Blend to Celestial Tripod in a clockwise motion to release constriction or blockages in the neck area and to encourage speaking your truth. This blend opens up the sinuses

---

[6] Andrew Ellis, Nigel Wiseman, and Ken Boss, *Grasping the Wind* (Brookline: Paradigm Publications, 1989), 52.
[7] Ellis, Wiseman, and Boss, *Grasping the Wind* , 52.

and stimulates the mind for clear thinking and for expressing ideas with confidence.

The fixed Earth nature of Taurus encourages holding on to material items and emotional wounds past their time. If you struggle with letting things go or are in a toxic environment, you may find your body storing toxins in nodules along the lower back, just above the crest of the hipbone (posterior superior iliac spine).

The large intestine organ alarm point, also known as, Large Intestine Shu, *Da Chang Shu*, Urinary Bladder 25, or UB-25, is found about one inch on either side of the spine at the level of the lower border of the spinous process of the fourth lumbar vertebra. When you follow this

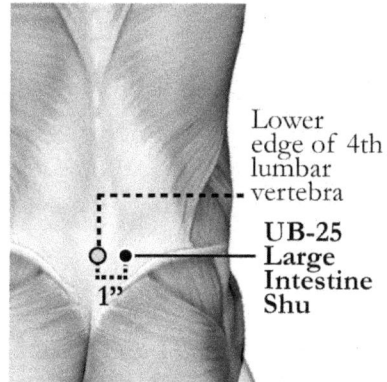

Lower edge of 4th lumbar vertebra

UB-25 Large Intestine Shu

1"

point out to the side of the body, you can feel the area where the body stores toxins in the nodules. In Chinese medicine, the *Shu* points support organ functions similar to the way chiropractors use specific spinal levels to alleviate the physical and emotional dysfunctions of the organ.

Applying a diluted Taurus Sign Blend to the lower back supports the healthy release of what is no longer needed physically and emotionally and safely breaks down fatty nodules in the area that store toxins.

Remember to dilute the Taurus Sign Blend if you have had excessive sun exposure, have sensitive skin, or are applying it to the lower back area around the large intestine alarm point. This blend is best used full strength when diffusing or when applying to the soles of the feet, where the skin is thicker.

Taurus Sign Blend Affirmations:	I am reliable and secure in myself. I am grounded and open to change. I hold on to what is of value and let go of what I no longer need.

The Gemini Archetype

The Energy of the Sign of Gemini and the Stomach Organ

Gemini, the Twins, is a mutable air sign. This is the time of year when we transition from spring to summer and when the pollinators (bees, butterflies, and hummingbirds) appear. The energy of Gemini mirrors the energy of the pollinators that move rapidly from flower to flower, appearing to enjoy the next flower as much as the one before.

With strong Gemini energy in your chart, you most likely love to take in new experiences and new learning. You enjoy making new connections and being social. You are likely a good communicator and enjoy conversation. In that the sign is associated with the image of twins, it also involves understanding and integrating different sides of yourself—the light and shadow or positive and negative aspects of who you are.

In balance, the energy of Gemini manifests as curiosity, good communication skills, and a strong rational mind. There is a love of learning and of exploring new ideas and gifts in networking with others. When worked consciously, it also involves being self-aware and actively integrating the different facets of your personality.

Out of balance, Gemini energy may be expressed as being scattered or gathering a lot of facts without integrating the knowledge. Being socially flighty and having difficulty engaging at a deeper level can be another manifestation of an out-of-balance Gemini. In addition, you may not feel fully integrated and may have inner conflicts with the different aspects of yourself.

The ruler of Gemini is Mercury, which is associated with the stomach meridian. The sign opposite Gemini, which helps it to be in balance, is Sagittarius. Sagittarius helps in seeing the "bigger picture." It also aids in processing information and understanding that information in a more integrated way.

In Western astrology, Gemini is physically associated with the shoulders, arms, hands, lungs, and nervous system. Under stress, injuries or problems in these areas may manifest.

In Chinese medicine, Gemini corresponds to the stomach organ, which controls the initial stages of digestion. The stomach organ works directly with several other organs, including the large intestine, spleen, pancreas, gallbladder, and small intestine to ensure proper digestion. When the stomach functions well, digestion is synchronized, and the organs that contribute to nourishing the body are harmonized. The spirit communicates effectively, and multitasking comes naturally. Both emotional stress and poor-quality foods can challenge the stomach organ and impair the entire digestive system. If your Gemini Sun, Moon, or Ascendant has challenging aspects, you may find yourself easily upset both physically and emotionally, both of which can be triggered by a variety of causes and can affect different aspects of the digestive system.

Key Themes for Gemini Sun, Moon, and Ascendant

GEMINI SUN:
If your Sun is in Gemini and you are working this in a conscious way, then you are most likely an extrovert who is comfortable conversing with others and enjoys learning from others as well as teaching. You have a good grasp of information and enjoy sharing your knowledge with others. You enjoy making connections with others and are effective in networking.

If your Gemini Sun is out of balance, you may have difficulty focusing your energy and tend to be active and always in motion and may even be hyperactive. You may love taking in new facts and new information but without integrating it or assimilating it in a meaningful way. You may get too bogged down in the analyzing the "trees" and lose the sense of the "forest" or bigger picture. You may enjoy connecting with others but have difficulty following through on the contacts, or you may tend to develop a lot of social connections without moving into deeper relationships.

GEMINI MOON:

With your Moon in Gemini, you may need to share and talk about your emotions with others. In this way, you deepen your own understanding of what you are feeling. Journaling is also a helpful way of engaging in self-dialogue and of deepening your awareness of your own emotions. It is most likely emotionally important to you to share and connect with others, and you are nurtured by being in groups and in social interactions.

If your Gemini Moon is out of balance, you may feel scattered and have difficulty tuning into your feelings on a deeper level. You may tend to talk over others or feel pressured to share your ideas and feelings without being very self-aware or taking in feedback from others.

GEMINI ASCENDANT:

With Gemini's energy on your Ascendant, you are apt to be seen by others as outgoing, engaging, and articulate. Others may see you as a good communicator or teacher, and you enjoy engaging with life through your ideas and your desire to make connections.

Out of balance, you may be scattered and go from activity to activity without a clear sense of direction or purpose. You may enjoy talking with others but lack emotional depth or an ability to fully integrate your own ideas or what you are learning from others. You may enjoy interacting with others but lack a sense of follow-through or commitment to deepening these relationships.

The Harmonizing Essence of the Gemini Sign Blend

The Gemini Sign Blend (also known as the Stomach Organ Supporting Blend) consists of 30% lemon (*Citrus limon*), 30% copaiba (copal: *Copaifera reticulate* or *Copaifera L. genus*), 30% patchouli (*Pogostemon cablin*), and 10% peppermint (*Mentha piperita*). The balancing nature of this blend effectively supports the duality of the sign of Gemini. The grounding effects of copaiba and patchouli and uplifting qualities of lemon and peppermint support Gemini's simultaneous need for stimulation and focus. Copaiba and peppermint are stimulating and cortisol boosting, while patchouli and lemon are relaxing and grounding. This blend also addresses the main components of a balanced immune system for long-term use.

In this blend, the intensity of patchouli is harmonized with the honey-like aroma of copaiba, the cleansing aroma of lemon, and the minty sweet aroma of peppermint. Most people find the patchouli in this blend appealing when combined with the other oils, thereby supporting the social nature of Gemini.

Patchouli's calming effect on both the nervous and digestive systems offer support for the occasional nervous stomach, the associated organ in Chinese medicine. Patchouli creates an energetic barrier to negativity in the environment, supporting emotional security; so, if you have a Gemini Sun, Moon, or Ascendant, you can embrace your social nature and find a safe setting to process more profound emotions.

Copaiba's stimulating and grounding properties give stable energy to fuel the need for stimulation and activity. Copaiba supports a healthy stomach lining and is easily added to drinks along with lemon and peppermint to quench your thirst for life. Lemon is generally uplifting and releases stagnation both physically and emotionally. Peppermint is cooling while it releases the build-up of heated thoughts that occur when Gemini feels stuck emotionally.

How to Use the Gemini Sign Blend

Diffusing this blend throughout the day supports your Gemini Sun, Moon, and Ascendant in its element (mutable air) by promoting healthy relationships and boosting energy. Applying the Gemini Sign Blend to the soles of the feet in the morning encourages direction, focus, and energy throughout the day. Diffusing or applying this blend as perfume is a quick reminder to relax and focus.

The acupuncture point Central Venter, also known as *Zhong Wan*, Conception Vessel 12, or CV-12, is the alarm point for the stomach organ. When the digestive system or the ability to make energy or *qi* is not functioning correctly, this point becomes tender or tight. Central Venter is found on the midline of the abdomen, midway between the umbilicus and the sternocostal angle (where the ribs meet and the xiphoid process begins). At birth, Central Venter is the first point that becomes active in the acupuncture meridian system and begins the flow of energy in the body, which then feeds into the lung meridian for the baby to take its first breath.

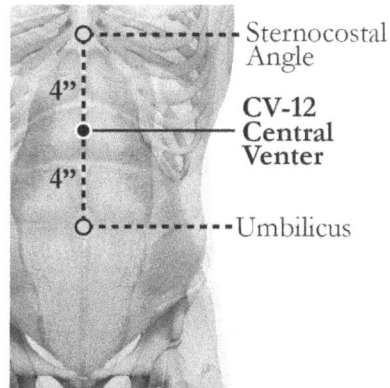

Central Venter harmonizes the *qi* or energy of the entire body and is the meeting point of the conception vessel with the small intestine, triple burner, and stomach meridians. Central Venter is the meeting and harmonizing point for all the yang organs, which includes the small intestine, large intestine, stomach, gallbladder, triple burner (lymph system), and urinary bladder. This busy point mirrors the busy lives of the Gemini Sun, Moon, or Ascendant.

Applying the Gemini Sign Blend to the midline of the abdomen will activate the Central Venter point to harmonize and energize the meridians that make up the digestive system. Start an inch above the point and rub the blend down to the belly button to support *qi* and energy production. Applying this blend clockwise over the point can keep ideas and action flowing to help you achieve your goals. Applying this blend in a counterclockwise motion can slow down an overactive digestive system and overactive mind to fully contemplate ideas. Adding the Gemini Sign Blend affirmations provides intention. You can repeat the phrases internally to create mantras and give the subconscious direction.

Gemini Sign Blend Affirmations:	I am centered and focused. I learn, grow, and pace myself. I connect and share with others in a thoughtful way.

The Cancer Archetype

The Energy of the Sign of Cancer and the Spleen and Pancreas Organs

Cancer, the Crab, is a cardinal water sign. This is the beginning of summer and the time when we experience the longest days of the year. The sign of Cancer relates to the archetype of the nurturing mother.

If you have a Cancer Sun, Moon, or Ascendant, you likely value your home and family life, and you naturally nurture and take care of others. The energy of Cancer also indicates emotional sensitivity and vulnerability. Like the Crab, you may need to keep a shell around your soft and tender heart.

When in balance, Cancer energy manifests as being nurturing, emotionally caring, sensitive, and valuing home and family.

Out of balance, Cancer can be expressed as neediness, insecurity, being emotionally "touchy," or being overly protective. It may also manifest as overextending oneself as a caretaker without factoring in personal needs and can even come across as "smothering."

Cancer is ruled by the Moon. It relates to our emotions and the experience of our bodies as well as to what nurtures us. The sign opposite Cancer is Capricorn, which helps to bring structure and a sense of responsibility to the sensitivity and emotionality of Cancer.

In Western astrology, Cancer is physically associated with the stomach, uterus, and breasts. Under stressful aspects or transits, if you have a Cancer Sun, Moon, or Ascendant, you might experience digestive or hormonal issues or problems with your uterus or breasts. You might also have difficulties in nurturing yourself.

In Chinese medicine, Cancer traditionally corresponds to the spleen organ, although it is generally accepted today to include the pancreas. The pancreas controls insulin production to stabilize blood sugar and releases a variety of digestive enzymes, most of which target digesting carbohydrates. The spleen supports the immune system and recycles red blood cells. When the spleen and pancreas are functioning optimally, the spirit feels nourished and energized, and the muscles are strong. Under stress, the immune system becomes depressed, and weight gain occurs primarily due to the stress hormone cortisol. If your Cancer Sun, Moon, or Ascendant has challenging aspects, you may find yourself struggling with weight gain and issues affecting metabolism, such as emotional eating, hypoglycemia or insulin resistance, or you may need to focus on strengthening your immune system.

Key Themes for Cancer Sun, Moon, and Ascendant

CANCER SUN:

If your Sun is in this cardinal water sign, and you are working with this archetypal energy in a conscious way, you are apt to be a caring and nurturing person who is sensitive to the feelings and needs of others. You are intuitive and emotionally responsive to what is going on around you. You value a stable and nurturing home life and make parenting or nurturing those that you love a top priority in your life.

If your Cancer Sun is out of balance, you may give too much to others emotionally without taking care of yourself and without honoring your own feelings and needs. You may get caught up in your own emotions and instincts and have difficulty seeing yourself or what is going on around you in a more rational or intellectual way.

CANCER MOON:

When working with the Cancer moon sign in a balanced way, you are in touch with your feelings and emotionally expressive. You are not likely to brood or hang on to resentments or strong feelings as you let the emotions flow through you and then pass on, like the waves on the surface of the sea. You are apt to be intuitive, perceptive, and caring in your relationships and interactions with others. You are very invested in parenting or being in a caretaker role with others.

If your Cancer Moon is out of balance, you may be moody and easily hurt. You may have difficulty balancing your own needs with those of others, especially family members, with a tendency to be overly giving or to have difficulty letting others be responsible for themselves. You are likely to be sentimental and emotionally reactive and lack an objective perspective on what you are feeling.

CANCER ASCENDANT:

With Cancer Ascendant, you are likely seen by others as a sensitive, caring, and nurturing person. You tune into others' feelings easily and express your own in an open way.

If your Cancer Ascendant is out of balance, you may be more introverted and hold yourself back in order to protect your feelings of insecurity or vulnerability. You may over-extend yourself emotionally or be seen as moody and overly sensitive.

The Harmonizing Essence of the Cancer Sign Blend

The Cancer Sign Blend (also known as the Spleen Organ Supporting Blend) consists of 40% tangerine (*Citrus nobilis* or *Citrus reticulata* var. *tangerine*), 40% fennel (*Foeniculum vulgare*), 10% clove (*syzygium aromaticum*), and 10% coriander (*Coriandrum sativum L.*). The nurturing combination of this blend supports both the physical and emotional needs to take in life to its fullest while feeling protected. The sign of Cancer is the caretaker in the zodiac and has a tendency to worry that there isn't enough to meet everyone's needs. The combined effect of these oils supports optimal digestion by aiding in nutrient extraction, strengthening the digestive tract lining, and assisting with healthy carbohydrate and sugar processing. This blend simultaneously addresses patterns of emotional eating.

Tangerine and fennel are two oils that are beneficial digestive aids for men and women. Tangerine is physically and emotionally uplifting to support a healthy metabolism and outlook in life. Fennel is prized for its ability to enhance fertility for both men and women by supporting a healthy reproductive system and balancing hormones. Fennel and tangerine also supply breastfeeding mothers with increased energy to take care of the needs of the home and family. Together, these oils provide a solid foundation for people to handle their emotional needs.

If you have a Cancer Sun, Moon, or Ascendant in your natal chart, you may feel the effects of the Moon's cycles and may find yourself especially sensitive to fluctuations in blood sugar throughout the day. Clove and coriander together stabilize sugar and carbohydrate processing to encourage constant solid energy and reduced sugar and carbohydrate cravings. Clove and coriander also support healthy bacterial flora to protect your body and digestive system from the environment.

All four oils in this blend encourage your body to adapt to your environment and immediate needs. With the properties of energizing and relaxing while nourishing and releasing, this blend will support you to take care of yourself and others in a balanced way and be prepared for any situation.

How to Use the Cancer Sign Blend

Diluting the Cancer Sign Blend and applying it to the entire abdomen in a clockwise rotation feels exceptionally nurturing. If your oils are approved for internal use, taking a few drops of this blend in a capsule with meals can help support a healthy digestive system and processing of sugar and carbohydrates in the diet. Diffusing this blend in the home creates a warm and nurturing environment.

The acupuncture point Great Embracement is a very important point that acupuncturists rarely use because it is too close to the lungs to needle. However, the close proximity to the lungs and other internal organs, along with the point's actions, make it ideal to use with essential oils.

Great Embracement, also known as Great Wrapping, *Da Bao*, Spleen 21, or SP-21, is found on the lateral line of the torso (the sideline) about six inches below the armpit. Sources differ in the

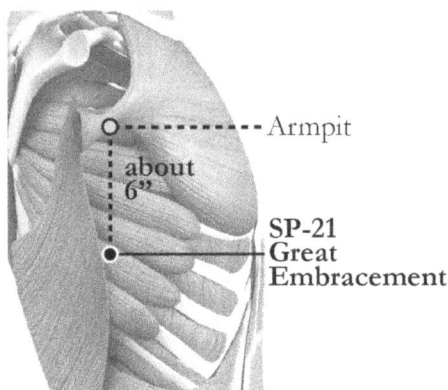

exact location and reference either below the sixth rib or below the seventh rib. Great Embracement is often tender and finding the sorest spot is the easiest way to identify this point.

Great Embracement is a special connecting point that harmonizes the internal organs and the yin and yang of the body. This includes the masculine and feminine traits, male and female hormones, and the left and right sides of the body. This point nourishes and energizes all the vital organs by improving the circulation of *qi* and blood. The sign of Cancer corresponds with the Moon, which can only be seen when it is reflecting the light of the Sun. The Great Embracement point helps you to find balance while relating to the outside world and close family members.

There are four different ways to apply the Cancer Sign Blend to Great Embracement. Applying this blend in a clockwise motion over tender areas will energize the point to promote nourishment for you and your internal organs. Applying it along the lateral line or sideline of the ribcage from about three inches above to three inches below the Great Embracement point will help you to have healthy boundaries and harmonize with your immediate environment. Applying the Cancer Sign Blend from the Great Embracement point forward to the front of the body encourages healthy relationships with women. And finally, applying it from the Great Embracement point backward to the back of the body encourages healthy relationships with men.

Caution: the Cancer Sign Blend contains tangerine, a citrus oil, and can increase sensitivity to sunlight. Clove oil is high in phenols and can irritate the skin when repeatedly applied in the same area. Remember to dilute this blend if you have sensitive skin or plan to use it long-term. You can customize the following affirmations based on the method you are using to stimulate Great Embracement. For example, the second affirmation can read, "I nurture the women in my life and also take care of myself" when applying the blend from the Great Enhancement point to the front of the body.

Cancer Sign Blend Affirmations:	I honor my sensitivity and pay attention to my needs. I nurture others and also take care of myself. I am able to give to others from a place of fullness within.

The Leo Archetype

The Energy of the Sign of Leo and the Heart Organ

Leo, the Lion, is a fixed fire sign. This is the hottest time of summer in the northern hemisphere. The energy of Leo is about the fire of creativity and self-expression. It manifests in the desire to shine and to be seen and recognized. It also relates to living from the heart and having the courage of a lion. In that

Leo is associated with the Sun, it also reflects a desire to seek enlightenment and to strive to live from the soul and in alignment with our divine purpose.

In balance, if you are a person with strong Leo energy in your birth chart, you are apt to be generous, big-hearted, and creative. Leo energy also often manifests in courage, passion, joy, and charisma. You are allowing the light and heat of the Sun and the expression of your true self to radiate light and warmth to others.

Out of balance, Leo can manifest in arrogance, self-centeredness, or self-absorption. This is when the ego becomes attached to the light being radiated as if we feel that the self is, in fact, the "Sun." The Leo energy out of balance can also manifest in a lack of passion or self-esteem.

The Sun is the ruler of Leo and is associated with the heart meridian. The sign opposite Leo, which helps it to be in balance, is Aquarius. Aquarius in opposition supports your passion and self-expression as a Leo, your desire to be of service to the community, and your ability to see life from a more analytical perspective.

In Western astrology, Leo is physically associated with the heart, and when under stress, you may experience heart issues.

In Chinese medicine, Leo corresponds to the heart organ. The heart propels blood, which contains your life-force, throughout the body and encourages your spirit to interact with the world. When functioning well, the heart organ beats at regular intervals and adapts to the changing needs based on your activity level. Both the body and spirit function best with routines that prepare you to be able to accommodate different physical and emotional terrains. If your Leo Sun, Moon, or Ascendant has challenging aspects, you may experience constitutional or genetic issues affecting the heart such as an irregular heartbeat or heart murmur.

Key Themes for Leo Sun, Moon, and Ascendant

LEO SUN:

When worked in a conscious way, if you have this fixed fire sign as your sun sign, you are most likely a passionate person who lives from the heart. You are charismatic and enjoy expressing your creativity. You are on a quest for enlightenment and want to share the light of love with others. You are generous and warm and enjoy affirming others. You see yourself as a vehicle for the Divine Light to move in and through you.

If out of balance with Leo Sun, you may suffer from feelings of insecurity and need recognition from others in order to feel a sense of self-worth. You may seek to be the center of attention in order to feel seen and to feel special. You may feel jealous or competitive with others who are in the spotlight and need continual affirmation and mirroring from others in order to feel confident.

LEO MOON:

When in balance, if you have a Leo Moon, you are warm, generous, and giving with others. You enjoy seeing others' gifts and affirming them. You live from the heart and are guided by your own passion and creative interests.

If out of balance with Leo Moon, you may "wear your heart on your sleeve" and be easily hurt if others do not see you clearly or misunderstand you. You may need external affirmation in order to feel emotionally secure and have difficulty maintaining a sense of emotional equilibrium or self-confidence.

LEO ASCENDANT:
With Leo Ascendant, you like making a dramatic appearance and enjoy wearing colorful clothes that draw attention to you. You are likely to be extroverted and outgoing and seen by others as warm and generous.

If out of balance with Leo Ascendant, you might find yourself focusing on attention seeking and recognition, and you may tend to have difficulty engaging with others in a more mutual and caring manner. You may be self-absorbed, seek to be the center of attention, and need others to see you as special.

The Harmonizing Essence of the Leo Sign Blend

There are two versions of the Leo Sign Blend (also known as the Heart Organ Supporting Blend) with different ratios. The first blend contains 40% marjoram (*Origanum majorana*), 40% cypress (*Cupressus sempervirens*), 10% neroli (orange blossom: *Citrus aurantium bigaradia*), and 10% helichrysum (*Helichrysum angustifolia* var. *italicum*). This first blend focuses on the emotional aspects of the sign of Leo and is highly beneficial for the skin. The second blend contains 30% marjoram, 30% cypress, 30% orange (*Citrus sinensis*), and 10% helichrysum. This second blend focuses on the physical aspects of the sign of Leo and has a citrus oil, which limits the application sites for this blend.

Both Leo Sign Blends support the heart organ, energize the muscles, benefit the cardiovascular system, and calm the nervous system. If you have a Leo Sun, Moon, or Ascendant, you may have natural leadership and networking abilities that these blends highlight, as mirrored by the heart muscle fueling the network of vessels that feed the body. In Chinese medicine, the heart organ stores your soul, and the three common oils support this function. If you have a Leo Sun, Moon, or Ascendant, you likely have a strong desire for action and for living out the soul's purpose with courage and passion.

Neroli in the first blend and orange in the second blend support the heart by uplifting and removing energetic blockages in the cardiovascular system. The aromatic properties of neroli oil are sensual and commonly found in aphrodisiac blends and perfumes. In ancient cultures, brides adorned themselves with neroli on their wedding day. Oranges are grown in regions of long daylight to take in energy from the sun and transform it into nutrients. Some, like d-limonene, are only found in its oil. Both neroli and orange foster Leo's connection to the Sun when their source energy feels depleted. Both oils can help you achieve your goals; neroli enhances emotional connections, and orange enhances physical action.

Marjoram essential oil both strengthens and relaxes healthy muscle tissue, which is beneficial since the heart is a muscle. Marjoram adapts to the immediate need of the heart to promote balance by simultaneously relaxing and strengthening the muscle tissue. Marjoram oil instills joy and a sense of immortality for the soul. This oil encourages your Leo Sun, Moon, or Ascendant to relax and enjoy life while experiencing your soul's journey.

Cypress circulates fluids and strengthens the cardiovascular system by targeting the veins and arteries. Cypress plays the role of messenger, helping your Leo Sun, Moon, or Ascendant transport your essence and life force to your immediate environment. This oil also releases blockages to help clear the way for Leo's self-expression and creativity. As an evergreen, cypress grounds and creates a feeling of security all year. Historically, cypress symbolized the cycle of life, death, and afterlife.

Helichrysum essential oil has a special chemical composition that adapts your blood flow to the ideal rate and viscosity for any situation and at any given time. Of all the oils, helichrysum has the most adaptability. The chemical constituents of helichrysum also promote a healthy nervous system to support the electrical conduction of the heart. Often the heart suffers more from imbalances due to the connecting nerves than in the organ itself. Helichrysum uplifts your subconscious to rise above barriers that are holding you back from expressing your soul's essence in this lifetime. This plant keeps its shape and fragrance long after harvest, which represents the soul's eternal nature.

How to Use the Leo Sign Blends

You can wear the Leo Sign Blend that uses neroli as perfume or use it diluted for facial rejuvenation. You may find applying this diluted blend especially helpful in improving skin texture and elasticity on the chest and neck from excessive sun exposure. You can also dilute a few drops of this blend per ounce of water in a glass spray bottle and spritz your face and chest throughout the day.

The Leo Sign Blend that uses orange is best diffused, applied to the soles of the feet, or applied to the spinal column. The orange oil will irritate skin that has experienced excessive sun exposure. Applying this blend to the soles of the feet will encourage you to take the next steps of your soul's journey. Having someone apply this blend along your spine (remember to stop below areas of sun-damaged skin on the neck) will harmonize your central nervous system and encourage connection to your higher-self. You can dilute either blend and apply to the following acupuncture points found in areas of reduced sun exposure.

The acupuncture point Cyan Spirit, also known as *Qing Ling*, Heart 2, or HT-2, is found on the inside of the upper arm about three inches above the elbow at the level of the heart. Depending on the source, the Chinese character *Qing* refers to a blue-green or cyan color that nourishes the heart, the deep red color of blood, the purple color of royalty, or a green color of sprouting plants that signifies new life. The Chinese character *Ling* refers to the feminine or yin aspect of the spirit stored by the heart. In Chinese medicine, the heart rules the body and is known as the supreme emperor. Cyan Spirit refers to the heart storing the sacred feminine aspect of the spirit or soul. Applying either Leo Sign Blend in a clockwise motion will energize and balance your masculine and feminine attributes.

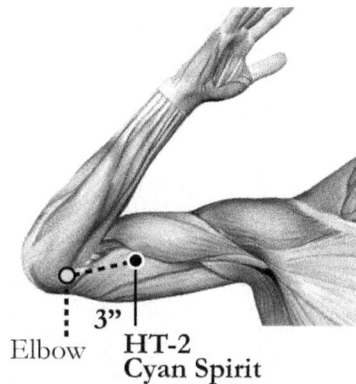

The acupuncture point Great Tower Gate, also known as *Ju Que*, Conception Vessel 14, or CV-14, is the alarm point for

Sternocostal Angle
2"
CV-14 Great Tower Gate

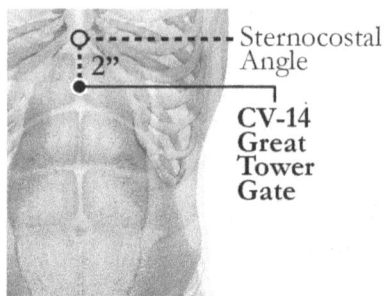

any disorder affecting the heart organ or the spirit. Great Tower Gate is found on the upper abdomen just below the xiphoid process, or two inches below the sternocostal angle where the ribs join. The ancient Chinese believed the xiphoid process resembled a gate to the chest cavity where the delicate lungs and supreme heart resided. If there was pain at this gate, then an imbalance was negatively affecting the physical or emotional aspects of the heart or spirit. Applying either of the Leo Sign Blends to this area in a clockwise motion will strengthen healthy boundaries and help clear imbalances negatively impacting your heart or spirit.

| *Leo Sign Blend Affirmations:* | I honor my inner fire and passion.

I radiate love and joy and express my creativity.

I live from the heart with courage. |

The Virgo Archetype

The Energy of the Sign of Virgo and the Small Intestine Organ

Virgo is related to the Harvest Goddess and is a mutable earth sign. It is associated with September and the fall harvest. Virgo's theme reflects living life with discrimination and discernment, being clear with priorities, and separating the wheat from the chaff. If you have a Virgo Sun, Moon, or Ascendant, you may demonstrate strong analytical and organizational abilities. These are ultimately skills to support you in discerning what is of value for yourself and for others. Virgo carries the energy of service, of commitment to health and self-improvement, and often is associated with healers.

When in balance, if you have strong Virgo energy, you have a good sense of your priorities and tend to live with discernment. You are likely to be organized and able to manifest what is important to you. You are focused on self-improvement and desire to be of service to others.

Out of balance with Virgo, you show a tendency to become overly focused on details or demonstrate a lack of discernment. Rather than using analytical skills for improvement and refinement, you may become overly self-critical or critical of others.

The sign opposite Virgo is Pisces. This helps balance your focus on daily life and on your physical and emotional health with your spirituality. Pisces in opposition gives Virgo a larger sense of meaning and purpose in order to stay clear about your priorities.

Mercury is the ruler of Virgo and relates to the mental abilities and organizational skills of people with this energy in their birth charts. Chiron is also associated with Virgo and relates to the healing aspects of this sign and the desire to use your gifts in the service of others.

In Western astrology, Virgo is physically associated with the small intestines and digestive system. If under stress, you may have digestive issues and have difficulties assimilating food.

In Chinese medicine, Virgo corresponds to the small intestine organ. In addition to its digestive functions, the small intestine produces a large number of neurotransmitters that affect mental and emotional health. Mental clarity and focused direction occur when the small intestine is functioning well. With stress, food allergies, or food intolerances, the small intestine struggles to process nourishment into the body, and the mind becomes clouded. If your Virgo Sun, Moon, or Ascendant has challenging aspects, you may struggle with sensitive digestion and mental fogginess.

Key Themes for Virgo Sun, Moon, and Ascendant

VIRGO SUN:

When worked consciously, the Virgo sun sign reflects a desire to be on a path of self-development and to be of service to others. You are likely to have a strong sense of discernment and discrimination and have clear priorities. You want to manifest your goals in a tangible way and are continually working on bettering yourself. You may be a healer or seek to benefit others with your gifts. You value the integration of body, mind, and spirit and want to live out your values with integrity in your daily life.

If out of balance with Virgo Sun, you may be overly focused on details, "missing the forest for the trees." You may also be so focused on the tasks in your daily life (your to-do lists) that you lose perspective regarding your priorities or what is of value in a larger sense. You also may be overly self-critical or critical of others, needing them to live up to your expectations and organizational standards.

VIRGO MOON:

With this moon sign, you are likely to be analytical with your emotions and seek to be on a path of self-development and growth. You value order and feel more secure when things are in their proper places. You analyze your daily patterns and seek to live a healthy lifestyle. You may take your diet seriously and be conscious and discerning about what is nurturing for you physically, emotionally, and spiritually.

When out of balance with Virgo Moon, you may be overly focused on details and on keeping things neat and organized in order to feel secure. If emotionally stressed, you may show some obsessive-compulsive tendencies. You also may tend to be overly critical of yourself, leaving you vulnerable to feelings of anxiety and a tendency to get caught up in obsessive thoughts. You may also be critical of others or tend to over analyze others' thoughts or actions.

VIRGO ASCENDANT:

With this mutable earth Ascendant, you are likely to be seen by others as grounded, analytical, and discerning. Your organizational gifts are valued, and you may be drawn to work that allows you to be of service to others.

If out of balance with Virgo Ascendant, you may be overly critical of yourself or others and get easily caught up in details or in the demands of daily life without being able to set priorities effectively. You may also have digestive issues or become anxious when under stress or if there is too much change or instability in your life.

The Harmonizing Essence of the Virgo Sign Blend

The Virgo Sign Blend (also known as the Small Intestine Organ Supporting Blend) consists of 30% marjoram (*Origanum majorana*), 30% copaiba (copal: *Copaifera reticulate* or *Copaifera L. genus*), 20% lavender (*Lavandula angustifolia*), and 20% lemon (*Citrus limon*). Virgo's dedication to sorting through life's experiences, in order to embrace that which is of worth and to discard the unworthy, is directly related to the small intestine's function of separating the clear from the turbid. With a Virgo Sun, Moon, or Ascendant, you may often find yourself enhancing others; the essential oils used in this blend enhance the properties of those they are blended with. The Virgo Sign Blend uses essential oils that can adapt their therapeutic properties, reflecting Virgo's mutable nature.

Supporting muscle tone and strength with marjoram essential oil allows the amino acid l-glutamine to focus on reinforcing the lining of the small Intestine. Marjoram essential oil also provides raw materials to help your Virgo Sun, Moon, or Ascendant get through your full schedule and busy workdays. Marjoram relaxes the muscles, at the same time strengthening them to encourage relaxation while working. Marjoram reduces excess stress hormones to foster a calm approach to sorting through stressful situations.

Copaiba boosts energy levels and concentration by supporting healthy cortisol output. When blended with other oils, copaiba enhances the properties of the other oils by adapting its therapeutic properties to complete the healing process. Copaiba encourages your Virgo Sun, Moon, or Ascendant to complete projects and make adjustments as needed for the greatest good of all involved. Copaiba's uplifting properties balance the relaxing qualities of marjoram.

When asked, "If you could only have one essential oil, which one would it be?" our response is lavender. Lavender's versatility supports Virgo's adaptogenic nature and its ability to handle every situation the user is presented with. The calming nature of lavender balances the uplifting properties of the lemon oil.

Lemon essential oil cleanses those aspects of life that do not serve your highest good, both physically and emotionally, to help release impurities as you discover them.

How to Use the Virgo Sign Blend

The synergistic blending of the two uplifting and energizing oils, copaiba and lemon, and the two calming and relaxing oils, marjoram and lavender, creates a balanced blend to use at any time of day. If your oils are approved for internal use, then a few drops in water or in a capsule with meals may support your digestive system. Diluting the Virgo Sign Blend and applying it clockwise over your abdomen will also support a healthy digestive system and the healthy sorting of ideas.

Applying the Virgo Sign Blend to the soles of the feet to start and end the day can help your Virgo Sun, Moon, or Ascendant process the details of the day on a subconscious level and while sleeping. This blend benefits the muscular-skeletal system, and applying it to the soles of the feet before or after workouts may enhance the benefits of exercise.

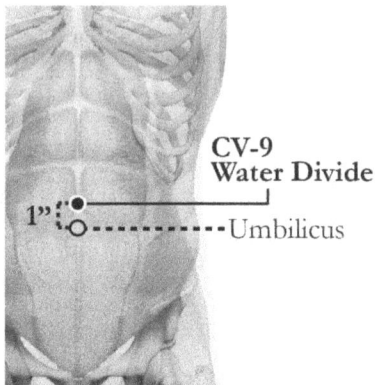

CV-9
Water Divide

1"

Umbilicus

The acupuncture point Water Divide, also known as *Shui Fen*, Conception Vessel 9, or CV-9, is found on the abdomen approximately one-inch above the belly button, the special point Spirit Gate. Water Divide becomes tight or tender when stress is too much for the adrenals to handle and specifically when stress is affecting the digestive system. Monitoring your Water Divide point is one way to know if your Virgo Sun, Moon, or Ascendant needs to make conscious changes to create a more balanced lifestyle. When applying the diluted Virgo blend to the abdomen, start with a few drops in Spirit Gate (the belly button) and circle outward, in a clockwise direction, around the belly button to include Water Divide. This will help you sort through stress and ground yourself to align with your higher-self and to work efficiently.

Virgo Sign Blend Affirmations:

I tend to the details in life in order to foster health and growth.

I see what is of value and cultivate what sustains me.

I analyze situations in order to be of service to others.

The Libra Archetype

The Energy of the Sign of Libra and the Urinary Bladder Organ Blend

Libra, the Scales, is a cardinal air sign. This is the time of the autumn equinox when the balance of light and dark is equal. The energy of Libra is about balance and harmony. It is also focused on mutuality in one-on-one relationships and the ability to be focused on the other's feelings and needs as well as our own. In a larger sense, the energy of Libra is also about wanting to be in right relationship (living with respect and care) in every aspect of life. It is about understanding the deeper meaning of balance and harmony and how this is the source of health in our own lives, in relationships with others, and in relationship with all of life.

In balance, Libra energy manifests in strong relationship skills, an ability for diplomacy, for seeing different perspectives and points of view, and the ability to foster mutuality and harmony in relationships. It is also often related to a love of art and beauty.

Out of balance, Libra may manifest in indecision or difficulties in relationships. Being overly analytical in relationships rather than relating from the heart or from compassion is another expression of a Libra when not in balance. It may also manifest in indecisiveness due to a tendency to see all points of view.

The planetary ruler of Libra is Venus, and this relates to how you are in relationship with others as well as your values and priorities in life. The sign opposite Libra is Aries. Aries in opposition helps you balance your ability to assert yourself and to be aware of your own feelings and needs with your sensitivity toward the feelings and needs of others.

In Western astrology, Libra is physically associated with the kidneys and lower back. When under stress, this may result in lower back pain or issues with the kidneys.

In Chinese medicine, Libra corresponds to the urinary bladder organ and the connections between the nervous system and the internal organs. The acupuncture points that control the urinary bladder organ are the farthest from the brain below the spinal column. When the urinary bladder function is compromised, it can be a signal that connections between the nervous system and vital organs need attention. When the urinary bladder is strong, the spirit feels connected to all vital aspects of life, which the other organs represent. If your Libra Sun, Moon, or Ascendant has challenging aspects, you may experience difficult or frequent urination and bladder control issues.

Key Themes for Libra Sun, Moon, and Ascendant

LIBRA SUN:

If you have the Libra sun sign and are working with it consciously, you value relationships and are attuned to others' feelings and needs as well as your own. You are likely to be diplomatic in your interactions with others and seek balance and harmony both interpersonally and in how you live your life. You may enjoy art and have a strong aesthetic sense.

If out of balance with Libra Sun, you may be overly focused on relationships and lacking in a strong sense of self or have relationship difficulties. You may also have difficulties making decisions and tend to over-analyze. You may have trouble accessing your deeper feelings and tend to look at things from a more intellectual perspective.

LIBRA MOON:

If you have your Moon in Libra and are living at a conscious level, you are able to attune to your own emotions and are sensitive to those of others. You value sharing thoughts and feelings with others in one-on-one interactions. You help others think through how to handle relationship issues and are a good mediator. You may love art and fill your home with works of art that foster a sense of harmony.

If out of balance with Libra Moon, you may over-analyze relationships and feel anxious about asserting yourself in interactions with others. You may be uncomfortable with conflict and tend to avoid difficult interactions. You may also feel indecisive and have difficulty knowing how to move forward if your feelings and needs conflict with those of someone you value.

LIBRA ASCENDANT:

With Libra Ascendant, you may be attuned to dressing in a way that shows your aesthetic sensibility and appreciation of beauty. Others are likely to see you as calm and balanced in how you interact and often turn to you to be a mediator or to handle conflicts with your diplomatic manner. You value fairness and strive to balance your needs with those of others.

If out of balance with Libra Ascendant, you may be overly accommodating in relationships and overly analytical. You may have difficulties accessing your deeper feelings or handling others' strong emotions. You may withdraw from conflict or have difficulties asserting your needs.

The Harmonizing Essence of the Libra Sign Blend

The Libra Sign (also known as the Urinary Bladder Organ Supporting Blend) consists of 25% ylang ylang (*Cananga odorata*), 25% geranium (*Pelargonium graveolens*), 25% clary sage (*Salvia sclarea*), and 25% blue spruce (*Picea pungens*). It is the only astrology blend that has equal parts of each oil. The combination of these four oils, in equal parts, perfectly balance each other to help Libra find balance in every aspect of their lives. Each oil in this blend targets a specific hormone pathway to support healthy hormonal balance for both men and women. Hormones interact closely with neurotransmitters, and the two together influence how you create emotional responses to the world around you. Ylang ylang's adaptogenic properties guide this blend to create balance between the male and female hormones for any person at any age.

The urinary bladder organ relates to the sign of Libra and depends on healthy nerve innervation from several different areas to work properly. The bladder receives signals from the vagus nerve, which is actually the longest pair of nerves in the body. The two main branches of the vagus nerve control the parasympathetic and sympathetic balance in the body. This balance controls a variety of activities such as rest and relaxation versus activity and alertness, and digestion and absorption of nutrients versus supplying energy to the extremities for movement. The bladder's nerve function also depends on the spinal nerves in the lower back. Because the bladder is one of the farthest organs from the brain, when the nervous system is out of balance or compromised, symptoms in the bladder are often the first to appear. The body is capable of repairing the nervous system; however, the raw materials needed to do this come from balanced hormonal levels.

The Libra Sign Blend supports healthy testosterone, progesterone, and estrogen levels for both men and women. Geranium has harmonizing properties to encourage proper blood flow, healthy liver function, and healthy bladder function. Geranium supports healthy pregnenolone and progesterone levels for both men and women. Geranium has historically been used to promote healthy menstrual cycles and emotional wellness. Surprisingly, geranium is also one of the best oils to use to keep annoying pests away and can help your Libra Sun, Moon, or Ascendant to know which people to let into your inner circle.

Clary sage is part of the sage botanical family and, unlike sage, it has a high amount of phytoestrogens (plant-based estrogens). Plastics and other chemicals found in the environment mimic estrogens in the body and clog the cellular receptor sites. Studies link xenoestrogens (synthetic-based estrogens) to both autoimmune diseases and reproductive cancers. Essential oils, in general, can help cleanse receptor sites, and clary sage, with high phytoestrogens, targets and cleanses the estrogen receptor sites. Clary sage has harmonizing properties to support healthy estrogen levels for both men and women and bladder function. Clary sage encourages the parasympathetic nervous system to relax and promotes restful sleep.

Blue spruce is part of the spruce botanical family and has a high amount of phytotestosterone (plant-based testosterone) to support nerve, muscle, and connective tissue regeneration. Blue spruce balances the female hormone properties of the geranium and clary sage in this blend. Healthy testosterone levels for both men and women stimulate action, motivate, and fuel will-power. Blue spruce can help your Libra Sun, Moon, or Ascendant overcome the tendency to indecision and inaction. The adaptogenic properties of ylang ylang allow the therapeutic benefits of this blend to shift and support the male and female hormones along with the yin and yang function of the body at any time of day or night.

How to Use the Libra Sign Blend

The harmonizing nature of the Libra Sign Blend makes it perfect to use any time you feel off balance. Diffusing this blend at night can help restore balance to the endocrine system and encourage restful sleep. Diluting the blend with a carrier oil and applying it along both sides of the spine and over the sacrum (the bladder meridian pathway) can help support the entire nervous system and balance the different hemispheres of the brain. Applying this blend undiluted to the soles of the feet will instill confidence in your decisions and encourage forward movement in your life.

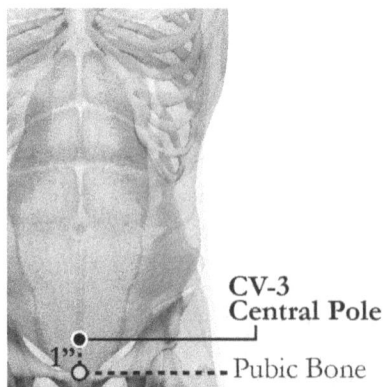

CV-3
Central Pole

1"

Pubic Bone

The acupuncture point Central Pole, also known as Middle Pole, Conception Vessel 3, or CV-3, is the front alarm point for the bladder organ, the meeting points of the conception vessel, and the yin meridians of the lower body: the spleen, liver, and kidney meridians. Central Pole is found on the front of the body about one inch above the pubic bone. Central Pole is the center point on the body for both the vertical and horizontal axis and the center point in the sky.[8]

[8] Andrew Ellis, Nigel Wiseman, and Ken Boss, *Grasping the Wind* (Brookline: Paradigm Publications, 1989), 306.

Applying the Libra Sign Blend, diluted with a carrier oil, in a clockwise motion over the acupuncture point Central Pole will bring grounding and balance for your Libra Sun, Moon, or Ascendant. This point balances the yin meridians, and when the yin is in balance, the yang naturally balances also. Central Pole is near the reproductive organs, which can benefit from the hormone-supporting oils in this blend. Applying this blend in a *counterclockwise* motion over Central Pole supports draining congested hormones and clogged receptor sites. Applying this blend in a *clockwise* motion over the reproductive organs is strengthening and nourishing.

Communication and choice of words are important for your Libra Sun, Moon, or Ascendant. Enhance this blend with the following Libra affirmations, or create your own affirmations to bring even more intention to your essential oil use.

| *Libra Sign Blend Affirmations:* | I am able to see my own and others' points of view.

I am committed to balance in relationships.

I am open to making changes to be fair to myself and others. |

The Scorpio Archetype

The Energy of the Sign of Scorpio and the Kidney Organ

Scorpio is symbolized by three images: the scorpion, the eagle, and the phoenix. Scorpio is a fixed water sign whose core theme is transformation. This sign includes those experiences (sex, death, deep emotions, trauma, etc.) that take us deep inside ourselves and encourage us to transform and to understand the cycles of life/death/rebirth. Depending on how we deal with them, we may become mired in the pain or intensity of these experiences and lash out at ourselves or others like the scorpion. We may try to rise above them and to hold a higher perspective like the eagle. Or we may go through a profound death/rebirth experience and emerge transformed like the phoenix.

In balance, the Scorpio energy shows the capacity to face intense experiences and deepen and grow through them. It manifests in emotional depth and intensity as well as the capacity to see and understand others at a deep level. If you have strong Scorpio energy in your chart, you may be unafraid of intense experiences and more likely to understand the deeper alchemical nature of these events or experiences and their ability to help you to grow and to find the "true gold" in yourself. You are also apt to be strong-willed, focused, and driven.

Out of balance, Scorpio energy may manifest as an abuse of power or a tendency to try to control others, or in highly negative experiences of trauma. It may also manifest in addiction to chaos or turmoil, or intensity for intensity's sake rather than for the purpose of transformation. You risk being self-destructive or vulnerable to becoming mired in depression, anger, or other negative primal emotions.

Pluto is the modern planetary ruler of Scorpio, and it relates to the intensity and transformational energy of this sign. The sign opposite Scorpio is Taurus, which helps the Scorpio intensity to stay grounded and to balance emotional depth with stability.

Physically, astrologically, Scorpio relates to the genitals, to the endocrine system, and to your capacity to regenerate and respond to stress (physically as well as emotionally). Under stress, you may show sexual difficulties, self-destructive tendencies, or autoimmune issues.

In Chinese medicine, the sign of Scorpio corresponds with kidneys, adrenals, ovaries, testes, and the brain. These organs determine your quality of life in your later years and how long your body can thrive on the physical plane. Your life force is your *jing* or essence, and the kidney organs store it. Your life force or essence stored in your kidney yin becomes the foundation for sexual and reproductive functions. Your life force or essence stored in your kidney yang warms the other organs and becomes the source of energy for movement, digestion, and transformation.

Key Themes for Scorpio Sun, Moon, and Ascendant

SCORPIO SUN:

If your Sun is in Scorpio and you are working with this at a higher vibrational level, you are likely to be intense, driven, and courageous. You are adept at dealing with crises and intense situations and see them as opportunities for transformation. You are able to face issues around death or transitions that others shy away from. In times of crisis, you have inner resources that allow you to move through a health or emotional crisis with a capacity to regenerate and recover rapidly.

If your Sun in Scorpio is not in balance, you may seek power or be in situations where either you are trying to have control over others or in situations in which you feel like you are the victim of a power imbalance. You may tend to see things as "black or white" and have strong reactions to situations or other people. You may get into situations that are intense and chaotic or self-destructive rather than transformational and empowering in a positive way.

SCORPIO MOON:

If your Moon is in Scorpio and worked with consciously, you are apt to be emotionally intense and may hold in your feelings, processing them internally. You are more introverted, have emotional depth, and courageously explore your own emotions. You are also able to read others well emotionally, being attuned to what is beneath the surface in your interactions with them. You are able to deal effectively with your own intense emotions, as well as with those of others, not fearing them but seeing them as important in the process of deepening self-awareness and inner healing and transformation.

If your Scorpio Moon is out of balance, you may be emotionally intense but tend to brood on your feelings or hold onto resentments or anger rather than working through them and using these as opportunities for increasing self-understanding or deepening relationships. You may deal with insecurities by attempting to control others. Or, you may handle stress in ways that are self-destructive or be vulnerable to periods of depression.

SCORPIO ASCENDANT:

With Scorpio as your rising sign, you are likely to be seen as introverted and emotionally intense. You are passionate and feel things deeply but tend to hold your feelings in and are selective about whom you really trust. Scorpio on the Ascendant usually indicates trust issues in relationships and requires that you work through your karmic or emotional issues around being vulnerable with others. If worked consciously, you will do your deep inner work in order to develop strong intimate relationships with others.

If not in balance, Scorpio Ascendant can manifest in your involving yourself in intense or traumatic relationships that reinforce your sense of mistrust. You may tend to stay in relationships that are turbulent, working too long and hard at trying to shift the relationship rather than getting clarity that it is an unhealthy situation and allowing yourself to disengage.

The Harmonizing Essence of the Scorpio Sign Blend

The Scorpio Sign Blend (also known as the Kidney Organ Supporting Blend) consists of 30% ylang ylang (*Cananga odorata*), 30% cypress (*Cupressus sempervirens*), 30% black spruce (*Picea mariana*), and 10% jasmine (*Jasminum officinale*). The synergistic combination and floral aroma of ylang ylang and jasmine soften the intensity, and sometimes the darkness that people under the sign of Scorpio can easily slip into. The black spruce and cypress provide depth of character that those with Scorpio crave. All four of these oils target the endocrine system and hormones, which strongly support emotional and mental health for processing the harder lessons your Scorpio Sun, Moon, or Ascendant often has to contend with.

In Chinese medicine, evergreens represent longevity in their ability to keep their leaves, remain green all year, and adapt to any weather condition. Your body stores your inherited and acquired essence in the kidneys, bone marrow, and brain, influencing your longevity. Acquired essence represents the energy added to your life force from your food, thoughts, and lifestyle. Chinese medicine uses tonics to increase acquired essence and classifies essential oils as the life force of the plant and the strongest of the tonics found in nature. Like the soul, evergreens are considered everlasting. They promote harmony by encouraging you to adapt to the environment and withstand the elements, or challenges, that life can bring. Ylang ylang is a tropical evergreen, cypress is a fast growing evergreen, and black spruce is one of the tallest evergreens.

Jasmine flowers, prized for their aroma and aphrodisiac properties, bloom only at night, requiring harvesting in the middle of the night to obtain the proper chemical makeup and aroma. In China, single jasmine "pearls" made from an individual flower open up in hot water to create an exquisite tea for special occasions. Jasmine essential oil provides a safe space for your Scorpio Sun, Moon, or Ascendant to open up and process the deep, and sometimes dark, feelings to transform and evolve your soul. Jasmine essential oil aids with women's reproductive health (ruled by Scorpio) and promotes uterine contractions, therefore, this oil should be avoided during pregnancy.

In Chinese medicine, ylang ylang's adaptogenic properties bring balance to masculine and feminine energy and male and female hormones. Ylang ylang can calm or uplift, and sedate or energize, which can help the fixed nature of your Scorpio Sun, Moon, or Ascendant to adapt to the current environment. Harvesting ylang

ylang flowers occurs at sunrise, symbolizing emergence from darkness to bring harmony and balance to our planet. Ylang ylang softens the raw emotions your Scorpio Sun, Moon, or Ascendant processes on a daily basis.

Cypress essential oil promotes circulation and the release of congested, backed-up fluids. The sign of Scorpio is a water element of a fixed nature; therefore if you are born with strong Scorpio influences, you may be predisposed to stagnant fluids and rigid emotions. Cypress encourages your Scorpio Sun, Moon, or Ascendant to release the past, forgive, and move on to bigger and better things in life.

Black spruce essential oil carries one of the highest vibrational frequencies in nature, thereby supporting with Scorpio to reach their highest potential. In the northern hemisphere, the black spruce reaches up to touch the aurora borealis, or Northern Lights, which some cultures believe are messengers from the heavens. Black is a color of protection in many cultures, and black spruce is a tree of protection for both our planet and all the creatures that dwell here. In many cultures, black is the color people wear to funerals symbolizing protection for the soul as it passes into the otherworld. In Chinese medicine, black is the color of the water element that represents the cycle of birth and death.

The three evergreens combined urge your Scorpio Sun, Moon, or Ascendant to lift your spirit to the highest level of consciousness and rise above your challenges while remaining true to your soul's purpose. The added jasmine softens the soul to find love and enjoyment on the earthly plane. Together these four oils offer your Scorpio Sun, Moon, or Ascendant a signature scent that evokes the senses at the deepest level, promotes self-confidence, and encourages the safe transformation of dark and hidden secrets. Your Scorpio Sun, Moon, or Ascendant can raise awareness for yourself and others of needed changes to improve the community and live a meaningful life.

How to Use the Scorpio Sign Blend

Diffusing the Scorpio Sign Blend at night supports transformation through the subconscious and dream state to help your Scorpio Sun, Moon, or Ascendant reach the deepest regions of your spirit energy. Wearing this blend as perfume during the day softens the harshness of the world to encourage taking risks and the next steps to support needed changes in your community. Adding a few drops of this blend to a cup of bath salts for an evening bath creates the ideal setting for your Scorpio Sun, Moon, or Ascendant to feel at home in your water element and to enhance meditation, visualization, or relaxation.

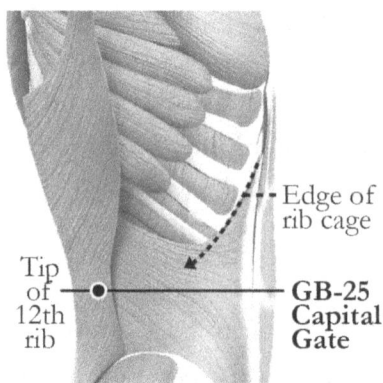

Edge of
rib cage

Tip
of
12th
rib

GB-25
Capital
Gate

The acupuncture point Capital Gate, also known as *Jing Men*, Gallbladder 25, or GB-25, is the front alarm point for the kidney organs. When the kidneys need attention, Capital Gate becomes tender, and on most people this point is tender because of dehydration. Capital Gate is found on the back, towards the side of the body at the free end of the last, or twelfth rib. The easiest way to find this point is to lie on your side and follow the edge of the ribcage down and back until you come to the final rib. Then follow this rib out to the side of the body until you find the end or tip of the rib.

The main action of Capital Gate is to harmonize the kidney and spleen organ functions of the body. When applied to astrology, Capital Gate's main action is to harmonize the deep and intense emotions felt by your Scorpio Sun, Moon, or Ascendant. Applying the Scorpio Sign Blend, diluted with a carrier oil, to Capital Gate will lighten the emotional weight carried by your Scorpio Sun, Moon, or Ascendant and help with forgiveness and releasing the stress of the day.

Scorpio Sign Blend Affirmations:	I align my will with Divine will.
	I dive deep into my feelings and re-surface with new insights.
	I seek true empowerment for myself and others.

The Sagittarius Archetype

The Energy of the Sign of Sagittarius and the Pericardium Organ

Sagittarius is a mutable fire sign. The image of Sagittarius is depicted as a centaur holding a bow and arrow, poised and ready to shoot. As the centaur, Sagittarius is half-human and half-horse; this image is also associated with Chiron and others in mythology who were wise mentors and teachers.

Sagittarius is the constellation that is close to our view of the galactic center, and the archer's arrow is pointed toward this place in the sky. In this way, Sagittarius reflects our search for Source and for meaning in our lives. Sagittarius carries the energy of the explorer, the seeker, the one who journeys within or travels the world in search of answers to the deeper questions of life. It reflects a longing to learn, not in an analytical way but in a more holistic and intuitive way. Sagittarius is about more right-brained ways of knowing and of integrating knowledge in order to see the bigger picture. The Sagittarian is more interested in gaining wisdom than in having knowledge.

In balance, strong Sagittarian energy manifests in enthusiasm for life and a love of exploration. It may be seen in strong philosophical or religious beliefs and in a strong sense of trust in the deeper purpose and meaning of events in life. It is the understanding that life is a journey of exploration and growth—spiritually, intellectually, and emotionally.

Out of balance, the energy of Sagittarius may manifest in travel for travel's sake or seeking adventure without utilizing the experiences for growth and understanding. It may be reflected in a lack of direction or a lack of spiritual beliefs. Or it may manifest at the other end of the spectrum as being overly rigid intellectually with dogmatic beliefs or religious fundamentalism.

Jupiter is the planetary ruler of Sagittarius and holds the expansiveness and exploratory nature of that sign. The sign opposite Sagittarius is Gemini. When in balance, Gemini in opposition supports the Sagittarian energy to express itself in writing, teaching, or dialoguing with others. This is the integration of learning with the longing for wisdom that leads to knowledge and your own beliefs about life.

Physically, astrologically, Sagittarius is related to the thighs and how we use our legs for movement. Under stress, Sagittarians may have difficulties with their hips or thighs or problems with the sciatic nerve.

In Chinese medicine, the pericardium organ protects the heart from infection, heat (inflammation), and unseen pathogens. It influences the esophagus and the initial stages of digestion, including the symptoms of nausea and vomiting (which in some instances occur along with heart attacks). When the pericardium meridian and organ are out of balance and compromised, logical and clear thinking is difficult. The pain referral areas for the pericardium include the chest and ribcage, shoulder and hip alignment, and the piriformis muscle that can cause sciatic nerve pain. The pericardium meridian strongly influences the production of blood, a woman's reproductive cycle, and the quality of her menstrual blood.

Key Themes for Sagittarius Sun, Moon, and Ascendant

Sagittarius Sun: If your sun sign is in Sagittarius and in balance, you are likely to have a strong sense of faith. You see life as a journey and enjoy learning and exploring ideas and cultural perspectives in order to deepen your understanding of life. You have strong beliefs that guide you, and you approach life in a philosophical and spiritual manner. You may be outgoing and enjoy sharing your knowledge and understanding with others through teaching or writing. You have an affinity for symbolism and metaphor and may be a good story-teller.

If your Sagittarius sun sign is out of balance or not worked at a conscious level, you may be rigid in your beliefs and insist that others adhere to your point of view. Or, you may lack a sense of direction and see life as an adventure without any deeper meaning or purpose. You may travel or explore the world for your own enjoyment without processing your experiences at a deeper emotional or philosophical level.

Sagittarius Moon: If your Moon is in Sagittarius and in balance, you love talking about the deeper questions of life and enjoy story-telling and sharing your wisdom with others. You love taking in new ideas and exploring other cultures in order to see life from differing points of view. You are passionate about your sense of life as a spiritual journey and are on a quest to integrate your own beliefs and understanding of life. You may also be optimistic, have a strong sense of faith, and enjoy interacting with others.

If your Sagittarius Moon is out of balance, you are likely to be extroverted and may enjoy social adventures and parties but have difficulty knowing your beliefs or having a focus in life. You are a good conversationalist and enjoy the stimulation of interacting with others but may not live at a spiritually conscious level. You may be a risk-taker or enjoy traveling and being in new situations for the stimulation rather than for the learning or deepening that you might gain from these experiences.

Sagittarius Ascendant: With this Ascendant, you may be an active and outgoing person who enjoys engaging in conversations with others about philosophical or spiritual issues. You may be a good conversationalist, teacher, or story-teller. Others may see you as charismatic and passionate or inspiring in your expression of your thoughts and beliefs. You may love to travel and explore the world both physically and intellectually.

If your Sagittarius Ascendant is out of balance, you may be adventurous but scattered, not having a clear sense of direction or purpose. You may seek external stimulation and have difficulty being alone. You may enjoy talking with others and sharing your ideas but lack a coherent sense of your own beliefs.

The Harmonizing Essence of the Sagittarius Sign Blend

The Sagittarius Sign (also known as the Pericardium Organ Supporting Blend) consists of 30% cedarwood (*Cedrus atlantica*), 30% copaiba (copal: *Copaifera reticulate* or *Copaifera L. genus*), 20% geranium (*Pelargonium graveolens*), and 20% cardamom (*Elettaria cardamomum*). With the job of protecting the heart and spirit, this blend releases inflammation, excessive heat, and stagnant fluids, along with keeping negative emotions and people away. When the environment is positive, and people are helpful, the soul's journey is pleasant and meaningful. This combination of oils promotes a clear head and movement of *qi* (energy), blood, and fluids to keep your Sagittarius Sun, Moon, or Ascendant focused and moving forward on your spiritual journey in life.

The combination of cedarwood and geranium is commonly used to keep bugs, ticks, and fleas away from people and four-legged friends. Ancient cultures around the world used cedarwood and geranium to ward off evil and protect houses and places of business. In the Sagittarius Sign Blend, they protect the spirit from troublesome people and create a protective aura for safe traveling and daily life. Cedarwood and cardamom are decongestants that cleanse hormone receptor sites and keep fluids flowing to prevent stagnation of old hormones, a condition that contributes to the restlessness you may experience if you have strong Sagittarius energy.

Cedarwood is high in sesquiterpenes, which supports and balances the endocrine glands in the head including the pituitary, hypothalamus, and pineal glands. Cedarwood's ability to harmonize and self-regulate allows it to adapt to the different needs of the body based on stress level, time of day, and environmental irritants. This supports the mutable nature of Sagittarius to adapt to any situation effortlessly.

Geranium has harmonizing properties for the blood that allows it to self-regulate its therapeutic properties and to support ideal viscosity and blood flow. Geranium has historically been used to support the aspects of the menstrual cycle that relate to blood flow. Geranium cleanses the blood and helps to cleanse negative emotions and keep your Sagittarius Sun, Moon, or Ascendant feeling optimistic.

Cardamom cleanses the cellular receptor sites, releases environmental toxins, and stimulates a healthy immune system response. Cardamom works with the lymph system to keep fluids flowing and the immune system to protect the borders of the body. Cardamom combined with geranium protects the heart and keeps harmful influences from affecting the spirit.

Copaiba is a resin that has high levels of sesquiterpenes and therapeutic properties that support a healthy inflammatory cycle for tissue repair and cellular regeneration in the brain. This combination supports clear thinking and focused direction for your Sagittarius Sun, Moon, or Ascendant. Copaiba naturally enhances other oils therapeutic benefits. In the Sagittarius Sign Blend, copaiba enhances the moving properties of cedarwood, geranium, and cardamom while providing a solid foundation and a grounded feeling.

How to Use the Sagittarius Sign Blend

Diffusing the Sagittarius Sign Blend at home creates a sacred space for your Sagittarius Sun, Moon, or Ascendant to feel safe and to release negative emotions and restlessness. Adding a few drops of this blend to cotton balls and placing them under the seats in your car provides energetic protection while keeping your car smelling fresh and clean.

The Sagittarius Sign Blend is slightly stimulating, and so applying it to the soles of the feet can help you start your day on the right foot to journey out into the world. Diluting this blend with a carrier oil or adding a few drops to a glass spray bottle and applying it before outdoor activities may help keep both pests and pesky people away.

The acupuncture point Chest Center, also known as *Shan Zhong*, Conception Vessel 17, or CV-17, is the front alarm point for the pericardium organ and the meeting point of the Conception Vessel and the spleen, kidney, small intestine, and triple burner meridians. Another name for this point is Original Child[9]; it personifies the youthful nature of the Sagittarius Sun, Moon, or Ascendant. Chest Center is found on the midline of the chest, over the sternum, at the level of the fourth intercostal space, in

---

[9] Andrew Ellis, Nigel Wiseman, and Ken Boss, *Grasping the Wind* (Brookline: Paradigm Publications, 1989), 320.

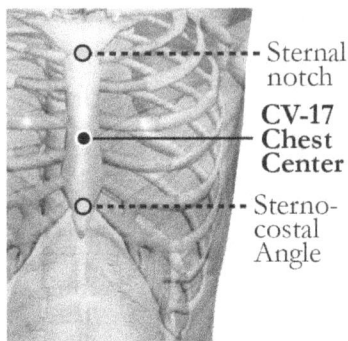

line with the nipples on men. This point is the approximate vertical midpoint between the sternal notch at the lowest border of the neck and the lower border of the xiphoid process.

Chest Center is also the meeting point for the *qi* (energy) of the body; the upper body is where the *qi* can become stagnant and congested. In Chinese medicine, *qi* strongly influences emotions and likes constant and steady movement. Applying the Sagittarius Sign Blend to Chest Center regulates the *qi* flow and increases the reserves. Chest Center is an active acupuncture point that becomes tender when any meridian is out of balance with the pericardium. When this point is tender, look for areas of your life that create imbalances for your Sagittarius Sun, Moon, or Ascendant. Applying the Sagittarius Sign Blend to Chest Center can help relieve frustration and promote clear thinking to keep you on your life path.

Sagittarius Sign Blend Affirmations:

I learn and explore
in order to understand
the deeper meaning of life.

I am focused on my
true path and purpose.

I live with faith and hope,
knowing that the sunrise
follows the darkest night.

The Capricorn Archetype

The Energy of the Sign of Capricorn and the Lymph System

Capricorn is a cardinal earth sign. The image for this sign is the "sea-goat." In ancient mythology coming from the Sumerian culture, the wise teachers came from the sea, from Source, in the form of fish and then changed into earth-creatures to bring their wisdom to the people. They taught the people how to farm, how to live on the Earth, and the ways of wisdom, and then they disappeared back into the sea. In this way, Capricorn in its essence is about leading and guiding others and bringing a sense of order to society.

In balance, Capricorn is about being responsible, living with good judgment and integrity, and striving to manifest goals that are of service to society. It also reflects living from an underlying sense of passion but knowing how to channel that in healthy ways.

Out of balance, Capricorn reflects a tendency to be bound by rules or tradition and to be overly focused on success. It may also manifest as emotional repression, or being overly tied to external expectations and your work or image in society. Or it can reflect living from your passion in an impulsive or out-of-balance way.

Saturn is the planetary ruler of Capricorn and shows in your astrological chart where you may feel challenged or bound by duty and yet also hold wisdom. The sign opposite Capricorn is Cancer. This supports you in integrating your sense of responsibility and duty with your emotions and in honoring the integration of your feelings and intuition with your actions in the world.

In Western astrology, Capricorn is physically associated with the skeletal system and the knees in particular. Under stress, Capricorns may have joint issues or problems with their knees.

In Chinese medicine, Capricorn corresponds to the lymph nodes. Hundreds of these are found throughout the torso, or trunk of the body. The lymph nodes connect with lymph vessels to support the immune system and filter toxins out of the blood. The lymph nodes store and mature lymphocytes that come from the bone marrow throughout the skeletal system. When the lymph nodes are functioning correctly, the body properly identifies and neutralizes environmental toxins, abnormal cells, and low-grade infections, and the spirit knows what influences are best to walk away from. Under stress, the lymph nodes struggle to protect the body. If your Capricorn Sun, Moon, or Ascendant has challenging aspects, you may experience swollen lymph nodes, swollen joints, immune system weakness, or challenges with releasing environmental toxins.

Key Themes for Capricorn Sun, Moon, and Ascendant

CAPRICORN SUN:
If your sun sign is in Capricorn, and you work this consciously, you are likely to be an ambitious, responsible, and hard-working person who longs to be of service in the world. You have natural leadership abilities, and you are effective at setting goals and pursuing them one step at a time the way a mountain goat reaches the top of the mountain. You like structure and organization and tend to set up clear plans in order to achieve your goals. You are attuned to societal systems and expectations and are aware of how to be successful within these structures. Beneath your responsible

and serious exterior, you may have an underlying passion that few realize is there.

If your Capricorn Sun is out of balance, you may be overly concerned with external rules and with pleasing those in authority, rather than being guided by your own inner wisdom or accessing your leadership skills. You may be driven to succeed but lose sight of the deeper nature of your sun sign which is about being of service through your gifts. You may also alternate between being overly responsible and then acting out with the underlying passion and wild side of Capricorn. Or you may be overly conscientious and concerned with following external rules and being compliant with authorities, but over time become increasingly reserved and depressed, losing connection with your passion and spirit.

CAPRICORN MOON:
With your Moon in Capricorn, you are likely to be emotionally reserved and may not easily connect with or express your emotions. You prefer to show restraint and to handle situations in a grounded and responsible manner. However, you may have moments when your passion surfaces, breaking through your guardedness.

If out of balance with your Capricorn Moon, you may have difficulties connecting with your emotions and tend to be overly serious and emotionally restrained. You may not know how to connect with others emotionally and may tend to be rule-bound and overly responsible. Or, you may vacillate between periods of being over-controlled emotionally with excessive, passionate outbursts.

CAPRICORN ASCENDANT:

If you have Capricorn as your rising sign and are working it consciously, you are responsible and adept at setting and achieving your goals. You like to have a plan, and then you are able to move forward in a decisive way. You like to be in charge of situations and show natural leadership skills. You are diligent and hard-working, and others see you as trustworthy and reliable. You are passionate and channel that in ways that are healthy for yourself and others.

If out of balance with your Capricorn Ascendant, you may be overly concerned with rules and overly compliant with external authorities, seeking to fit in with conventional societal norms. You may be anxious in unstructured situations or when the expectations of you are not fully clear. You tend to be overly serious and "buttoned up" rather than relaxed and at ease in your life and with others. You may have periods of passionate expression following by guilt and regret.

The Harmonizing Essence of the Capricorn Sign Blend

The Capricorn Sign (also known as the Triple Burner Organ Supporting Blend) consists of 30% cedarwood (*Cedrus atlantica*), 30% balsam fir (*Abies balsamea*), 30% hinoki (*Chamaecyparis obtusa*) and 10% ledum (*Ledum groenlandicum*). These four essential oils come from slow-growing, mature trees or plants and carry with them the ability to survive. All four of these oils support the healthy aging of the skin, bones, and connective tissue. All four of these oils have cleansing and immune boosting properties that target the lymph system.

Most mature trees continue to grow in the center, hidden from the world. When you see them on a daily basis they look the same; however, with the passage of time, they are clearly achieving their goals. Tree bark resembles aging skin and protects the tree from unwanted attention, infections, and harsh weather. If you have a Capricorn Sun, Moon, or Ascendant you likely value these properties and the longevity found in these evergreens.

Cedarwood has adaptogenic properties that change its therapeutic benefits based on the environment, stress level, and time of day used. Cedarwood can help your Capricorn Sun, Moon, or Ascendant adapt to different stressors while remaining cooperative and flexible. Cedarwood supports healthy brain development for children and adolescents and preserves brain function in the elderly; times in life when being flexible and adapting to changes in daily routines can be challenging. Cedarwood is a choice wood for construction because it is highly stable and doesn't change shape due to humidity or weather, and it resists fungus, microorganisms, and insects.

Fir trees are evergreens that are commonly farmed in the Americas for Christmas trees to celebrate the birth of Jesus, which occurs during the sign of Capricorn. Mature fir trees provide shelter in nature due to their dense needles and pyramid shape. Fir essential oils are restorative and transform stress and nervous tension in the form of cortisol into fuel for regeneration. Because of the adaptive nature of cedarwood, either balsam or white fir (*Abies grandis* or *Abies concolor*) is acceptable to use in this blend.

Hinoki, sometimes referred to as Japanese cypress, is the preferred type of cypress in this blend because it is a high-quality wood. It is often used in fine Japanese construction, such as temples, churches, and other buildings used for gatherings. If hinoki is unavailable, cypress (*Cupressus sempervirens*) is an acceptable substitute. Hinoki essential oil is more relaxing and calming than its cypress counterpart, however, both support the lymph system, circulatory system, and fluid movement throughout the body.

Ledum is part of the rhododendron family, and Labrador tea is made from the leaves. The leaves are also used to make the essential oil; they are slow-growing and harvested annually. Both the tea and the essential oil are strong, so small doses are optimal for therapeutic effects. Ledum is cleansing and stimulating and targets the lymph nodes, which are critical to the immune system and tissue regeneration. The lymph system is the adaptive portion of the immune system that allows your body to remember how to fight off most infections.

Your body generates adult stem cells in the lymph system for tissue regeneration and healing. With age, your ability to generate these cells declines and healing becomes more challenging. The regenerative properties of the evergreen trees, combined with ledum, creates a blend you can rely on for longevity and stability. Your Capricorn Sun, Moon, or Ascendant will find the earthiness of its aroma comforting and the grounding effect stabilizing for emotional health.

How to use the Capricorn Sign Blend

Your body heals and regenerates at night while you sleep. Therefore, diffusing the Capricorn Sign Blend at night will enhance the regenerative qualities of the blend. Applying this blend to the soles of the feet in the morning will help your Capricorn Sun, Moon, or Ascendant feel grounded and adapt to unforeseen changes in your life. Everything applied to the skin absorbs into the lymph system, and by adding a few drops to an unscented, non-toxic lotion base, you will support your lymph system and create a protective barrier like the bark on the trees. You can apply this blend to any area of congested lymph nodes.

The acupuncture point Celestial Well, also known as *Tian Jing*, Triple Burner 10, or TB-10, is the earth point on the triple burner meridian that corresponds directly with the lymph nodes. Celestial Well is found on the back of the arm about one inch above the tip of the elbow in a hollow created between the tendons and the bone with the arm slightly bent. The epitrochlear lymph node is found at the Celestial Well acupuncture point.

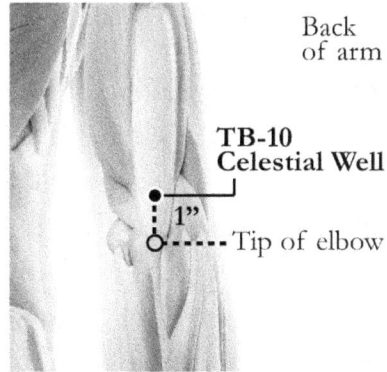

The triple burner meridian is a fire meridian that governs the waterways in the body. The ancient description of Celestial Well is a small pond surrounded by high cliffs. Another meaning of this name is the courtyard in certain styles of Chinese houses.[10] Both of these meanings highlight material structures created from the Earth. Applying the Capricorn Sign Blend to Celestial Well can help you bring structure and a solid foundation to ensure your goals have longevity. Because this point is a celestial point, it will also calm the spirit and help you connect with your higher self to make sure you're focused on your spiritual path.

The acupuncture point Window of Heaven, also known as *Tian You*, Triple Burner 16, or TB-16, is the original "Window of

---

[10] Andrew Ellis, Nigel Wiseman, and Ken Boss, *Grasping the Wind* (Brookline: Paradigm Publications, 1989), 239.

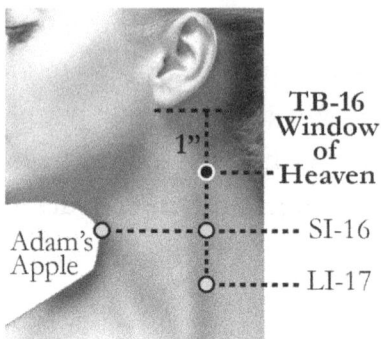

TB-16
Window
of
Heaven

1"

Adam's
Apple

SI-16

LI-17

Heaven" point that gave five points on the neck special status as access points for the heavens. The Window of Heaven group of points controls rebellious and chaotic energies that rush to the head causing headaches, dizziness, sudden onset of deafness, and swelling of the face. Window of Heaven is found on the side of the neck, behind the larger neck flexor muscles, about one-inch below and behind the base of the ear. The Window of Heaven group of points is found near the large numbers of lymph nodes on the neck. Applying the Capricorn Sign Blend, diluted with a carrier oil or lotion, to the side of the neck will target absorption into the lymph nodes to promote clear and focused thinking, dispersing rebellious and chaotic energies.

Capricorn Sign Blend Affirmations:

I follow through on my goals in a flexible manner.

I honor my passion as well as my sense of responsibility.

I am guided by wisdom and inner knowledge.

The Aquarius Archetype

The Energy of the Sign of Aquarius and the Gallbladder Organ

Aquarius, the Water-bearer, is a fixed air sign. The image of the Water-bearer is of the person who is pouring the urn of living waters to the Earth. Aquarius is about understanding that everything is energy, and everything is interconnected. The "living waters" and flow of energy foster all that is and connect and support all of us. Aquarius is reflected in analytical abilities and good skills in understanding organizations and societal systems. If you have strong Aquarian energy, you may be a reformer, pioneer, or visionary who strives for a better, more just and fair world.

In balance, Aquarian energy manifests as strong analytic skills, a capacity to see things from a larger perspective and a passion for justice and equality. It reflects an openness to diversity, a valuing of what is true and meaningful rather than adhering to illusions or traditional ways of doing things. As an Aquarian, you likely show a strong capacity for independence, and you desire freedom for yourself and others. You are often uncomfortable in hierarchical dynamics and rebel against misuse of power.

Out of balance, Aquarian energy may manifest as being detached or aloof from personal relationships. It may also be expressed in rebelliousness and a sense of alienation or of not feeling understood or able to fit into society. It can manifest in a fear of change.

Uranus is the modern planetary ruler of Aquarius and reflects the unconventional energy of Aquarius and the commitment to truth and justice. The sign opposite Aquarius is Leo. The Leo energies support balanced living from the heart in a personal way with the passion for social issues and concerns. It helps to integrate the analytical side of Aquarius with personal warmth, creativity, and self-expression.

Physically, astrologically, Aquarius relates to circulation, to the nervous system, and to the ankles. Under stress, Aquarians often show problems with the nervous system or problems such as fibromyalgia or circulation issues. They may also have a vulnerability to sprained ankles or other ankle injuries.

In Chinese medicine, the gallbladder organ relates to the sign of Aquarius. The gallbladder governs decision making and clear thinking. The gallbladder organ makes bile for the proper digestion of fats and promotes collagen production to support healthy bones and connective tissue. When the gallbladder organ is not functioning optimally, fats are not properly digested, and the body cannot complete a normal and healthy inflammatory cycle, generate hormones, or fuel the brain. Genetically modified foods and oils in today's diet burden the gallbladder and create health challenges if you have weak gallbladder function.

Key Themes for Aquarius Sun, Moon, and Ascendant

AQUARIUS SUN:

If your sun sign is in Aquarius and you are working this at a higher vibrational level, you are likely to be concerned with societal issues and value justice and fairness. You may be a pioneer or reformer, trying to improve society through your actions. You tend to approach life analytically and strive to see the bigger picture. You may be somewhat emotionally detached due to this more intellectual approach to life, but you want your life to be of service to society, and you value friendships, community, and shared goals. You enjoy being in group situations and have a good understanding of group dynamics and systems.

If your Aquarius Sun is out of balance, you may be emotionally detached and have difficulty getting close to others. You may be overly focused on societal reform and on your larger goals, without showing sensitivity to others or having good interpersonal skills.

AQUARIUS MOON:

With Aquarius as your moon sign, you tend to analyze your feelings and may have difficulty allowing yourself to be vulnerable or to connect easily with your own or others' deeper emotions. You are apt to be uncomfortable with emotional outbursts. You value justice, are sensitive to abuse of power, and are accepting of others in their diversity. You enjoy being in groups and being part of a community.

If your Aquarius Moon is out of balance, you may be rebellious and uncomfortable with external rules or authorities. You value justice but may become reactive if you feel mistreated or see others as not being treated fairly. You may also have difficulty being aware of your emotions or allowing yourself to be vulnerable. You tend to care more about social issues than about individual people.

AQUARIUS ASCENDANT:

With this rising sign, you are likely to be seen as extroverted and are drawn to being a part of a group or community that shares your values and social concerns. You want to make a difference in the world; you have strong social values and want to be an advocate for justice, equality, and fairness.

If your Aquarius Ascendant is out of balance, you are likely so committed to your social causes that you do not allow yourself to deepen emotionally or know how to relate to others in a vulnerable and intimate way.

The Harmonizing Essence of the Aquarius Sign Blend

The Aquarius Sign (also known as the Gallbladder Organ Supporting Blend) consists of 30% lavender (*Lavandula angustifolia*), 30% marjoram (*Origanum majorana*), 20% rosemary (*Rosmarinus officianalis*), and 20% wintergreen (*Gaultheria procumbens*). This combination balances the stimulating properties of rosemary and wintergreen with the relaxing qualities of lavender and marjoram to create an energizing and grounding blend useful anytime during the day. The essential oils in the Aquarius Sign Blend support healthy gallbladder digestive functions, help thin congested gallbladder bile, and encourage normal regeneration of the muscles and connective tissue of the body.

If you have an Aquarius Sun, Moon, or Ascendant, you may be prone to circulation issues and stress, which can manifest as issues with blood pressure. Lavender and wintergreen benefit people with hypertension or high blood pressure and rosemary benefits people with hypotension or low blood pressure. Marjoram can regulate and normalize blood pressure. Used together, these oils adapt to stress response and blood pressure fluctuations to help your Aquarius Sun, Moon, or Ascendant manage the life force flowing throughout your body.

Rosemary, marjoram, and lavender are members of the mint botanical family and support healthy digestion and immune functions. Wintergreen is a member of the Ericaceae botanical family, which includes a variety of plants that grow in acid soil, keep their leaves green all year, and have berries. The wintergreen essential oil in this blend comes from the Gaultheria species because of its mint-like aroma. Wintergreen oil breaks up congestion in the body and supports healthy digestive and immune functions.

The Aquarius Sign Blend supports emotional and mental health to help your Aquarius Sun, Moon, or Ascendant process ideas and stay calm while making a stand for beneficial change and long-term growth for humanity. Lavender calms the mind and promotes feelings of unconditional love. Marjoram promotes happiness and going with the flow. Rosemary releases old negative patterns to allow for new ideas and habits to form. Wintergreen stimulates the mind and provides mental endurance to stick with long-term goals. Together these oils provide energy and a positive outlook for your Aquarius Sun, Moon, or Ascendant.

How to Use the Aquarius Sign Blend

Diffusing the Aquarius Sign Blend during the day promotes clear thinking. Apply it to the soles of the feet in the morning to start the day off on a positive and uplifting note. Applying this blend, diluted with a carrier oil or non-toxic unscented lotion, along the spine can balance and regulate the central nervous system.

Applied diluted over the right side of the ribcage it can harmonize the liver and gallbladder for improved function.

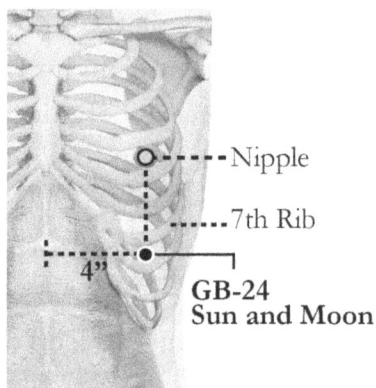

The acupuncture point Sun and Moon, also known as *Ri Yue*, Gallbladder 24, or GB-24, is the front alarm point for the gallbladder and the meeting point of the gallbladder and spleen meridians and the Yang Linking Vessel. Sun and Moon is found on the front of the rib cage, about four inches to either side of the midline, vertically in line with the nipple, and below the seventh rib.

The point name "Sun and Moon" reflects how this point harmonizes the yin and yang energies of the liver and gallbladder organs. Sun and Moon represents Aquarius's dual nature as an air sign that bears water. This is also a meeting point of yin and yang meridians. This point facilitates clear thinking. Another name for this point is Spirit Light, which speaks to the task of enlightening humanity which Aquarius holds dear.[11]

In Chinese medicine, the right side of the body is the yang side and the left side is the yin side. Applying the Aquarius Sign Blend in a clockwise rotation on Sun and Moon on the right side of the ribcage will support the physical attributes of the gallbladder organ. Applying the Aquarius Sign Blend in a clockwise rotation on Sun and Moon on the left side of the ribcage will support more of the emotional aspects of the gallbladder and Aquarius archetype.

---

[11] Andrew Ellis, Nigel Wiseman, and Ken Boss, *Grasping the Wind* (Brookline: Paradigm Publications, 1989), 273.

Aquarius
Sign Blend
Affirmations:

I see the bigger picture.

I honor my commitment
to truth and social justice.

I manifest my higher purpose.

The Pisces Archetype

The Energy of the Sign of Pisces and the Liver Organ

Pisces, the Fish, is a mutable water sign. The image for this sign depicts two fish swimming in different directions, yet tied to each other, joined at the "sacred knot." The meaning of Pisces revolves around having a strong yearning for connection with Spirit, with other realms or altered states of consciousness, while also needing to know how to be here on the Earth. Pisces energy is about understanding the oneness of all that is and the compassion that arises from that unity of consciousness. It is about wanting to live from love and in service to a mission or vision larger than oneself.

If you are in balance with strong Piscean energy, you likely have a strong mystical or spiritual nature. You may be creative, artistic, or have musical interests or abilities. You long to dissolve the boundaries of ego and the constraints of the mind to open to other ways of consciousness. You have high ideals, and you live a life of service or sacrifice, rather than living out of self-interest. You are intuitive, empathic, and compassionate.

Out of balance with Pisces, you may seek altered states of consciousness through drugs, alcohol, or other addictions. You may lose your boundaries and become emotionally overwhelmed, losing a clear sense of self and possibly becoming either caught in illusions or even psychotic.

Neptune is the modern planetary ruler of Pisces and reflects the energy of dissolving boundaries, strong intuitive gifts, compassion, and the longing to be of service. The sign opposite Pisces is Virgo. Virgo grounds the vision and expansiveness of Pisces, and it helps provide a balance and focus to the sensitivity and intuitive nature of Pisces.

Physically, astrologically, Pisces relates to the lymph system, sensitivities to external pathogens, or auto-immune issues. Under stress, Pisceans may manifest unusual symptoms, diffuse pain, or have systemic, chronic medical problems that are hard to define or diagnose. In addition, Pisces imbalances may manifest in addictions or liver problems. Pisces also relates to the feet, and if you have a Pisces Sun or Moon, under stress you may have foot problems or difficulties with balance or with staying grounded.

In Chinese medicine, the liver organ corresponds with the sign of Pisces, and most physical or emotional imbalances include a liver imbalance. Imbalances affecting the liver can stem from exposure to toxins, drug or alcohol use, or improper diet. Often, other not-so-obvious causes are compromised liver function, environmental sensitivities, genetic issues, inability to detox, exposure to heavy metals, chronic low-grade pathogenic infections, allergies and food intolerances, or overuse of prescription medications.

From a spiritual perspective in Chinese medicine, when your intuition or connection to your Source (divine guidance) is strong, it is easier to live your soul's purpose in this lifetime. When your connection to your Source is weak or out of balance, overcoming challenges with a self-empowering attitude and staying on your path becomes more difficult. When you feel your faith or connection to your Source wavering, it may mean the liver organ is out of balance.

Key Themes for Pisces Sun, Moon, and Ascendant

PISCES SUN:

With Pisces as your sun sign, and if worked in a conscious way, you are likely to be sensitive and intuitive, with a longing to be of service to something larger than yourself. You may be invested in doing work that is spiritual in nature or involves charitable or caretaking work of some kind. You have a natural mystical nature and enjoy expanding your consciousness through meditation, music, or other healthy ways of accessing altered states of consciousness.

If your Pisces Sun is out of balance, you may be a dreamer, having difficulty feeling grounded or accomplishing your goals. You may struggle with personal boundaries and tend to try to blend in with others. You may also seek to "dissolve" yourself or expand your consciousness in unhealthy ways such as through drugs or alcohol.

PISCES MOON:

If Pisces is your moon sign, and if worked at a high vibrational level, you are likely to be intuitive, empathic, and compassionate.

You are emotionally and psychically sensitive and tend to tune into what others are feeling easily. You have a good imagination and are likely to be mystical or spiritual. You may have vivid dreams and an ability to tune into guidance from other realms.

If your Pisces Moon is out of balance, you may have difficulty separating your feelings from those of others around you and have trouble maintaining personal boundaries. You may easily get flooded by emotions and then feel vulnerable and overwhelmed. Under stress, you may seek to escape through drugs or alcohol, or by disappearing into your imagination, or get caught up in illusions.

PISCES ASCENDANT:

If Pisces is your rising sign, others likely see you as sensitive, compassionate, and caring. You are likely to be empathic and emotionally open with others. You are giving and strive to be of service in your relationships and in the world.

When Pisces Ascendant is out of balance, you may have boundary issues emotionally or interpersonally, or you may get into dynamics where you are the caretaker or victim in interaction with others. You may have difficulties asserting yourself and may feel taken advantage of by others. You are likely to be more introverted in nature, and you may feel sensitive to external stimuli and need alone time in order to center yourself and tune into your own emotions.

The Harmonizing Essence of the Pisces Sign Blend

The Pisces Sign Blend (also known as the Liver Organ Supporting Blend) consists of 40% fennel (*Foeniculum vulgare*), 40% orange (*Citrus sinensis*), 10% rosemary (*Rosmarinus officianalis*), and 10% celery seed (*Apium graveolens*). Together these oils support optimal liver health to both release stored toxins and prevent imbalances from arising when exposed to environmental, personal, and emotional toxins in the future. Building a strong foundation for the liver and a secure connection to Source is the best way to prepare your Pisces Sun, Moon, or Ascendant for life's challenges in good times and challenging moments.

Fennel belongs to the parsley family, which includes some of the strongest and safest detoxifying plants. Fennel supports the digestive system, which is responsible for safely transporting toxins out of the body, and reduces detoxification symptoms, including a bad taste in the mouth, upset stomach, and irregular bowel movements. Fennel also supports the kidneys, the other organ of detoxification. Fennel essential oil is beneficial for any type of infection in the digestive system due to its universal anti-pathogenic properties. Fennel's detoxification properties target xenoestrogens. These substances are found in plastics and are causing many of the estrogen-dominant conditions plaguing the hormonal balance of both men and women.

Citrus essential oils, like orange, support the liver by providing enzymes needed for the detoxification process, and they support the digestive system by strengthening the digestive tract lining to transport the toxins out of the body safely. Citrus fruits grow in climates with abundant sunshine (the Earth's energy source) and can support your secure connection to your Source. Of all the citrus oils, orange essential oil has the strongest harmonizing properties to help your sensitive Pisces Sun, Moon, or Ascendant adapt to every environment and safely process toxins, toxic people, and hidden stressors.

Rosemary essential oil is high in the chemical constituent known as 1.8 cineol, a robust cellular cleanser and protector. Rosemary essential oil works best in small amounts to provide your Pisces Sun, Moon, or Ascendant a layer of protection and encouragement to leave behind people and attitudes that are not in alignment with your highest good and connection to your Source. When used in large amounts or long-term, rosemary essential oil can increase blood pressure if you have high blood pressure or a family history of hypertension. In this case, you can substitute clove essential oil in this blend.

Celery seed and fennel essential oils both have intense aromas; however, when blended together they harmonize and soften each other. Celery seed is a strong liver supporting oil that releases stored toxins and liver congestion. Celery seed, like fennel, also supports the kidneys and assists in the safe release of toxins from the body. Celery seed has relaxing properties to help calm your Pisces Sun, Moon, or Ascendant sensitivities and promote restful sleep and peaceful dreams.

How to Use the Pisces Sign Blend

Diffusing the Pisces Sign Blend helps to create a feeling of sanctuary in your home to release the day's stressors, cleanse the mind, and strengthen your connection to your higher self or Source. This blend also cleanses and purifies the air to support a healthy immune system. If your brand of essential oils is approved by the FDA for internal use, a few drops of this blend in a capsule taken with meals will support a healthy digestive system and the release of toxins that burden the body. Diluting this blend with a carrier oil and applying it over the right side of the rib cage will support healthy liver function and harmonize the liver with the digestive system.

The acupuncture point Cycle Gate, also known as *Qi Men*, Liver 14, or LV-14, is the alarm point for the liver organ and the intersecting point for the spleen and liver meridians and the yin linking vessel. Cycle Gate is found on the front of the rib cage about four inches to either side of the

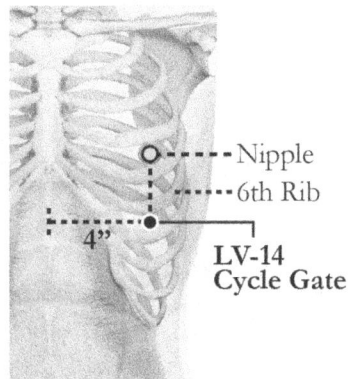

midline, vertically in line with the nipple, and below the sixth rib. This point is also directly above the Sun and Moon acupuncture point. Cycle Gate on the right side of the rib cage becomes tender with a congested liver or when the liver organ is out of balance.

As Pisces is the last sign of the zodiac, Cycle Gate is the last point on the acupuncture meridian system and completes one full cycle of the energy almanac in Chinese medicine. The connecting point on the lung meridian, Cloud Gate, shifts energy in the meridian system from Pisces to Aries as is most active at 3 a.m. The use of the term "Gate" indicates that this point provides access for your spirit energy or *qi* to enter and exit the acupuncture meridian cycle.

Applying the Pisces Sign diluted with a carrier oil at Cycle Gate helps to detoxify the blood and release unwanted emotions. Applying this blend to Cycle Gate before meals supports the digestive system and gently stimulates the detoxification process. Applying this blend to Cycle Gate before bed encourages the subconscious to release negative emotional habits that hinder your Pisces Sun, Moon, or Ascendant on your spiritual journey through this lifetime.

| *Pisces Sign Blend Affirmations:* | I am deeply connected with Spirit.

I trust my intuition and tune into my inner guidance.

I honor my dreams and am grounded in my reality. |

The Journey to Higher Vibrational Living

Love one another and help others to rise to
the higher levels, simply by pouring out love.
Love is infectious and the greatest healing energy.

—Sai Baba

We have followed Allie in her journey of using the astrology oil blends, working with her astrology chart, and utilizing Chinese medicine to make significant changes physically, emotionally, and spiritually in her life. Across the year of working with this energy healing process, she resolved her hormonal imbalances, skin issues, and physical fatigue. Her depression cleared, and she felt more engaged in her relationships. She also gained clarity about her more profound path and purpose in life, and how she could manifest her gifts in the world in a way that felt more in alignment with her true self.

The changes in Allie led to improvements in her relationships with her husband, family, and friends. Her community now sees her as a role model for transformation and for living life from a sense of being true to herself and her purpose. In living at a higher vibrational level, her life is filled with more joy and purpose and has a profound effect on those around her. She now finds herself sharing with others how to use the astrology essential oils to experience a life of fulfillment and authentic self-expression.

This journey of transformation, healing, and raising your vibrational level can be yours also. Through working with this integration of astrology, Chinese medicine, and essential oils, you can come into balance physically and emotionally, discover your true self, and feel empowered to live your life with a sense of purpose and higher consciousness.

As you deepen your understanding of your sun sign and your Sun's planetary aspects, you will understand more fully the light and gifts of who you uniquely are. You will also begin to experience your daily connection with the Sun and its healing and empowering energy. You will become more consciously attuned to the rhythms and energies of the seasonal cycle. Using the Transiting Sun Luminary Blend, you can work with the daily and seasonal energy of the Sun to raise your vibrational level and be in alignment with the natural energies around you. Through understanding the energies of your sun sign and the meridians and organs associated with this sign, you grow in awareness of your strengths and vulnerabilities; this then enables you to regain balance and use the essential oils and planetary and sign affirmations to function at your highest potential.

As you gain more awareness of your moon sign and the planetary aspects to your Moon, you become more conscious of who you are emotionally and how to deal with your feelings and the rhythms of your body. You feel more attuned to the energy of the lunar cycle and how to honor the aspect of the cycle that you were born into and resonate with. Living in a higher vibration and being more in balance with your body and emotions and the energies of the lunar cycle allows you to feel more at peace and more in harmony with yourself and with others.

Being in balance and living from a higher vibrational level allows you to live out the fullness of your gifts and to thrive in your life. You then become a light and inspiration to others, and you can support others in finding healing, balance, and empowerment to live their purpose and be their authentic selves.

Let us join together in this journey of healing, of coming into balance, of living at a higher vibrational level, and in attunement to the energies of the natural world and the cosmos. Astrology and Chinese medicine give us keys to the strategies for living in balance with ourselves and with the energies of the Earth and the cosmos. The astrology essential oils open the door to healing and transformation, and the planetary and sign affirmations help us to integrate these changes and manifest our highest potential. Let us all begin this journey of healing and transformation now—for ourselves, for our communities, and for the world.

The Healing History of Astrology, Chinese Medicine, and Essential Oils

The Origins of Astrology

Astrology is the oldest known art and science, woven into the ancient wisdom traditions of most cultures. For example, astrology is a core part of the Ayurvedic wisdom and healing traditions of India. Modern Western astrology finds its foundation in the ancient Egyptian and Mesopotamian use of the energies of the stars as a tool for healing and spiritual initiation. Healers and philosophers of ancient Greece and Rome further cultivated the application of astrology, and this knowledge was spread to healers and sages around the world.

At its essence, astrology is the understanding that everything is energy, and everything is interconnected. Quantum physics indicates that we reside in a holographic universe; by attuning to the energies of the stars and planets, we gain access to an understanding of the core themes and patterns unfolding on the Earth and in our own lives. The patterns of the stars and planets show how the energies of the times are affecting us individually and collectively.

Modern Western astrology (horoscopic astrology) originated in ancient Mesopotamia (now modern Iraq). Beginning in ancient Sumer, around 3,000 BCE, we see the origins of writing. These early cuneiform texts were star omens, referred to as the *Enuma Anu Enlil*. Another collection of omens was the Venus tablet of Ammizaduga related to the phases of Venus. Over subsequent centuries, the ancient Babylonians continued to observe the sky and developed a more complex understanding of the solar and lunar cycles (including the eclipses) as well as the movements of the planets. These sky omen texts formed the first phase of astrology.

The original Mesopotamia zodiac had only six signs, and time was recorded in cycles of sixty. In our current modern zodiac, these configurations are separated into twelve signs. We see this same pattern of six signs in ancient China, and there is a direct correlation between the original Chinese and Babylonian names of the constellations. Historians believe that Chinese astrology originated in Babylon and was brought to China around the sixth century BCE. In this ancient form of the zodiac, the current constellations of Aries and Taurus were seen as part of the Bull. Cancer and Leo were known as the Lion, while Virgo, which is one of the largest constellations in our modern system, was seen as the Harvest Goddess. The stars of Libra were viewed as claws and were fused with Scorpius forming the Scorpion. Sagittarius and Capricorn were known as the Goat-Fish, and Aquarius and Pisces together formed the Fish-Man. These ancient zodiac wheels began with the stars of Pleiades (in the sign of the Bull, now modern Taurus) on the eastern horizon. This makes sense given that these early zodiacs were developed when the stars of the Bull (Taurus) were rising at the time of the vernal equinox, marking the Age of Taurus.

Many ancient cultures were sophisticated in their understanding of the stars and how their energies were mirrored on the Earth. The ancient Egyptians as well as ancient cultures in Peru, Mexico, Old Europe, and other parts of the world aligned buildings and sacred sites with certain stars. Many of these sites were configured to mark the energies of the constellations or of the Sun at the time of the solstices or equinoxes. These practices were designed to align the Earth with the sky, bringing the energies into balance, harmony, and right relationship, which these ancient cultures knew was critical for their health and well-being. Many of the standing stones at ancient sacred sites were also carefully positioned along certain ley lines (energy lines on the earth) to balance or harmonize energies, much like acupuncture needles on the body's energy meridians.

Later, in the second phase of astrology (about 630 to 450 BCE), the more modern zodiac developed, consisting of the twelve signs along the ecliptic. These signs tracked the movement of the Sun throughout the year. The energy of the Sun through the seasonal cycle affected the rhythms of life on Earth, timing in agriculture, and the qualities of those born in each phase of the annual cycle. These twelve signs were also important in Jupiter's orbital cycle of twelve years. Jupiter would move through one sign of the zodiac each year. This was particularly important in Chinese astrology which to this day continues to mark each year with the sign of the zodiac that Jupiter is in during that year.

The third phase of astrology was the development of the horoscope or birth chart by the late Babylonians, known as Chaldeans, around 410 BCE. At that time, they began to analyze what signs the planets were in as well as the Sun and Moon, in order to assess how these energy patterns would influence the Earth and those born at a particular time. This was the starting point of the birth chart that continued to be developed in ancient Greece and Rome and has evolved into what we now use in modern Western astrology.

In modern Chinese astrology, the focus is on the birth year (e.g., being born in the year of the Wood Sheep) but also incorporates the energies of the date and hour of birth. This relates to the synthesis of the Chinese Energy Almanac and the ten heavenly stems and twelve earthly branches, which are considered to link the energies of the Earth and sky and seasonal cycles.

It is important to note that the current modern Western tropical zodiac, used to cast the birth chart, sets the wheel of the year and seasonal cycle as they were at the time of these first horoscopes. They were developed in the Age of Aries when the stars of Aries were rising at the time of the spring equinox. This is why the astrological wheel of the year begins with Aries, marking the spring equinox, and then continues around the wheel counter-clockwise. The modern tropical zodiac tracks this seasonal cycle, marked by the equinoxes and solstices, and no longer synchronizes with the actual positions of the constellations in the sky.

The constellations have shifted in their relation to the equinoxes and solstices since the origins of the first horoscopes. This is due to the process of precession, which occurs because of the tilt of the Earth's axis and other factors; so that from our perspective, the sky seems to shift backwards one degree every seventy-two years.

Since the astrological wheel of the year was established in the Age of Aries, the sky has "shifted" twenty-three degrees. This means that the signs and the constellations are no longer fully synchronized. For example, now when you are born under the sign of Aries, the Sun is actually in the stars of Pisces. The signs of the modern Western astrological wheel are actually marking the energies of the seasonal cycle and the cycle of the Sun through the course of the year, and no longer indicating the Sun's actual placement in the stars in the sky.

This seasonal movement goes around the wheel of the chart in a counterclockwise way. However, we track the diurnal cycle (the movement of the Sun, Moon, and planets in the sky over the course of a day) in a clockwise manner. This correlates with how we watch the Sun, Moon, and planets rise in the east and move clockwise across the sky to the west. These different cycles are important to remember as we look at the connections between Western astrology, traditional Chinese medicine, and the acupuncture meridian system.

A Brief History of Western Medical Astrology

Western medical astrology is rooted in ancient Mesopotamia; it flourished during the time of ancient Greece through the work of Hippocrates and Galen. Astrology was as an adjunct to medicine and provided an understanding of times of vulnerability to illness, the expected course and duration of diseases, and the best approaches to treatments. Understanding the planetary rulers of the signs and the signs' associations with different energies and atmospheric conditions assisted in guiding healers and physicians in how to address health issues.

In ancient Egypt, India, and China, as well as Greece and Rome, imbalances leading to illness were considered to be related to the four humors. This concept was developed in depth by Hippocrates, who lived from 460 to 370 BCE. The bodily fluids, or humors, were associated with personality traits or temperaments. The four humors were related to the four elements as well as different atmospheric conditions. The four humors were: sanguine (air—hot/moist), melancholic (earth—cold/dry), phlegmatic (water—cold/moist), and choleric (fire—hot/dry). The planetary associations with different weather conditions paralleled the development of the meridian system in traditional Chinese medicine, which was also related to the elements and atmospheric conditions.

For the ancient Chinese, the primary constellations were the Green Dragon in the east (associated with the wood element), the Red Bird in the south (fire element), the White Tiger in the west (metal element), and the Black Tortoise or Snake in the north (water element). The center was China itself (earth element).

The correlations between these four Chinese constellations and the Western zodiac are:

Green Dragon (wood element):   Virgo, Libra, Scorpio
Red Bird (fire element):   Gemini, Cancer, Leo
White Tiger (metal element):   Pisces, Aries, Taurus
Black Tortoise/Snake (earth element):   Sagittarius, Capricorn, Aquarius

Since ancient times, herbal remedies were used for medicinal and healing purposes. Plants were associated with atmospheric properties (hot, warm, neutral, cool, and cold) through their flavors (spicy, bitter, sweet, sour, salty, and bland) and were identified with particular planets. This association of plants, planets, and different energies continued through history and appeared in such well-known works as *Culpeper's Complete Herbal*, by the English botanist, herbalist, and physician Nicholas Culpeper (1616 -1654). It also mirrors traditional Chinese medical theory.

Also dating from ancient India and ancient Greece was the concept of the "doctrine of signatures," which held the understanding that the shapes, colors, and properties of plants resembled their healing properties and their associations with certain planets and with various parts of the body and the emotions that they helped to treat. For example, yellow flowering plants were associated with the Sun and could be used to treat depression; white flowering plants that grow in moist environments were identified with the Moon and might be used to treat women's menstrual problems.

Modern Western astrology no longer depends on the concept of the humors, but it does continue to draw on the associations of planets with plants, with the energies of the elements, and with atmospheric and seasonal conditions. While arising from different roots, both modern Western astrology and traditional Chinese medicine track the parallels between the energies of the seasons, atmospheric conditions, planetary energies and the associated symptoms of emotional and physical imbalances. Both astrology and Chinese medicine hold the understanding that the energies of the sky are mirrored in the energies on the Earth and in the human body. "As above, so below."

Despite these close correlations, however, the two systems differ somewhat in their understanding of health issues. From the Western astrology perspective, the signs of the zodiac correlate primarily with the physical aspects of the body, from Aries at the head to Pisces at the feet. Western astrology is more symptom-focused while Chinese medicine is more focused on the interconnectedness of the body and its energy systems.

In general, the bio-energetic and emotional aspects of the meridians and organs correlate more closely with the archetypal meanings and energies of the planets and signs rather than the physical attributes. The chart below summarizes the major correlations between Chinese medicine meridians and the Western astrology ruling planets, along with their associated medical functions or physiological and bio-energetic processes.

Correlations between Chinese Medicine Meridians and Planetary Rulers of Western Astrology Signs

	TCM Meridian	Western Astrology Planet
	Lung	**Mars (ruler of Aries)**
Function:	Controls breath, energy, pulse, blood	Blood, energy
Emotions:	Self-esteem	Self-confidence
Out of Balance Emotions:	Grief, shame, anxiety	Insecurity, low self-esteem
	Large Intestine	**Venus (ruler of Taurus)**
Function:	Release of toxins through intestines and bowels	Metabolic processes, insulin, assimilation of sugar
Emotions:	Balanced energy	Grounded, stable, sense of self-worth
Out of Balance Emotions:	Apathy, depression, irritability	Feeling stuck, difficulty letting go
	Stomach	**Mercury (ruler of Gemini)**
Function:	Nourishment through digestion	Autonomic nervous system, brain
Emotions:	Grounded, in balance	Clear thinking, calm
Out of Balance Emotions:	Affects mental state; confusion, hyperactivity	Anxiety, hyperactivity, feeling scattered

	TCM Meridian	Western Astrology Planet
	Spleen	**Moon (ruler of Cancer)**
Function:	Assimilation of nutrients, quality of fluids in the body	Fluids in the body, digestive process
Emotions:	Sense of balance, harmony	Emotionally stable, caring
Out of Balance Emotions:	Worry, obsessions, memory issues	Memory issues, overly emotional
	Heart	**Sun (ruler of Leo)**
Function:	Controls mind and emotions, houses the spirit	Core sense of self, essence, vital energy
Emotions:	Love, joy	Love, strong sense of self
Out of Balance Emotions:	Guilt, hate, longing, craving	Poor sense of self, low energy
	Small Intestine	**Mercury (ruler of Virgo)**
Function:	Assimilation of nutrients and emotions	Intestinal activity
Emotions:	Discernment, good judgment	Analytical skills, discernment
Out of Balance Emotions:	Agitation, confusion	Self-critical, judgmental of others
	Urinary Bladder	**Venus (ruler of Libra)**
Function:	Storage and excretion of urinary wastes, autonomic nervous system	Senses, balance of sugar and insulin
Emotions:	Balance, harmony	Balance, harmony
Out of Balance Emotions:	Fear, jealousy	Poor interpersonal skills
	Kidney	**Pluto (ruler of Scorpio)**
Function:	Core reservoir of energy	Internal process, endocrine system
Emotions:	Wisdom, self-understanding	Wisdom, self-understanding, insight
Out of Balance Emotions:	Insecurity, loneliness	Insecurity, intimacy issues

	TCM Meridian	Western Astrology Planet
	Pericardium	**Jupiter (ruler of Sagittarius)**
Function:	Protects the heart	Growth functions
Emotions:	Sense of joy, pleasure	Expansive feelings, faith, wisdom, confidence
Out of Balance Emotions:	Instability, emotional outbursts	Lack of faith, difficulties with self-confidence
	Triple Burner	**Saturn (ruler of Capricorn)**
Function:	Regulates transportation and transformation of system, fluids, and nourishment	Skeletal system
Emotions:	Kind-hearted, sense of peace	Grounded, stable, wise
Out of Balance Emotions:	Guilt, instability	Guilt, rigidity, fear
	Gallbladder	**Uranus (ruler of Aquarius)**
Function:	Stores and secretes bile	nervous system, assimilation of oxygen
Emotions:	Courage, drive, initiative	Initiative, pioneering spirit, clarity
Out of Balance Emotions:	Timid, indecisive	Fearful of change, rebellious
	Liver	**Neptune (ruler of Pisces)**
Function:	Growth, development, stores blood	Lymphatic system
Emotions:	Compassion, kindness, creativity	Compassion, creativity, sensitivity
Out of Balance Emotions:	Anger, resentment	Delusions, insecurity, overly-sensitive

The Healing History of Traditional Chinese Medicine

Traditional Chinese medicine remains the oldest continually practiced healthcare system in the world, used by over 25% of the world's population for over 3,000 years. The ancient sages developed the fundamental principles in such a way that they adapt to changes in disease, technology, or lifestyle and integrate well with other healthcare systems. There are eight treatment approaches referred to as the Eight Branches of Traditional Chinese Medicine. These include acupuncture, herbalism (including essential oils), medical massage, astrology, nutrition, exercise, genealogy (environmental influences), and meditation. All Eight Branches use the same system of energy circuits in the body, called acupuncture meridians, as their fundamental basis. The ancient healers believed in knowing and using all Eight Branches to promote a healthy lifestyle.

The acupuncture meridian system consists of a network of twenty channels (twelve main meridians and eight extraordinary vessels) that move energy in a rhythmic pattern throughout the body. The eight extraordinary vessels develop first at conception and guide the earliest separation of cells that form into the various systems of the body such as the respiratory, circulatory, endocrine, reproductive, nervous and digestive systems. These extra vessels direct the distribution of energy (*qi*) and blood throughout the body.

The twelve main meridians flow in a twenty-four-hour circuit with each meridian peaking for a two-hour period. The main meridians pass through different layers of tissue, from the skin through the connective tissue, muscle, bone, and organs. During the two-hour peak time, the organs related to those meridians are most active and the symptoms that occur during that time of day are often associated with an imbalance in the respective meridian.

In ancient Chinese culture, people honored their ancestral lineage by making concerted efforts to heal and to improve upon any genetic weaknesses (ancestral *qi*) they believed could be passed down to future generations. Before birth, the life-force of the unborn baby remains active in the eight extraordinary vessels and controls the developing meridian system, which becomes active at birth. Ancient Chinese culture looked at pregnancy as a special time. Friends and family assisted with duties expected of the pregnant women to lessen physical and emotional stress, so the future generation had the best health possible.

When the baby is born and takes its first breath, the ancestral *qi* activates the meridian system and begins to circulate through the body in the order of the Chinese meridian clock. For the first few weeks after birth, the baby's meridian system will acclimate with the diurnal rhythms of the mother's meridian system. During this sacred postpartum time, the mother was not separated from her baby, so they could both heal and balance to the proper meridian flow. If a baby became agitated or colicky during a specific two-hour period on the meridian clock or at the transition time, then the baby or the mother's corresponding meridian was out of balance.

The plant and animal substances used for medicinal purposes by the ancient Chinese physicians differed greatly depending on whether they were treating the emperor or the common folk. The Chinese emperors obsessed over longevity to extend their reign, and essential oils, known as the *jing* or essence of the plant, contained the life-force that would add to the emperor's energy reserves.

In the 1920's the communist party came into power and deemed acupuncture and traditional Chinese medical theory as inferior and actively discouraged the practice of it. The oral traditions and ancient Chinese medical secrets for extending longevity for the emperors and their families were lost along with most of the ancient medical texts. Therefore, traditional Chinese medicine practiced today lacks the original references to essential oils. However, Michelle blends ancient Chinese medical theory with modern essential oils and clinical applications to embrace today's emerging energy medicine.

The Healing History of Essential Oils

Ancient cultures depended on medicinal plants for healing and survival. Plant remains are found in Neolithic graves indicating the use of plants in funeral rites and the possible use of plants for healing. The oldest written evidence of the use of plants as medicine was found in a Sumerian clay tablet dating to around 3,000 BCE. In it were recipes for plant preparations involving over 250 different plants including poppy, henbane, and mandrake.

Shamans, the medicine men and women of indigenous cultures, believed that by communicating directly with plants, they were able to discover the plant's medicinal value. The shamans thought that plants had consciousness, and developing a relationship with the spirit of the plant enhanced its healing energy. Even in modern times, researchers seek the knowledge of shamans and indigenous people to gain more understanding of the medicinal value of various plants. Most pharmaceutical medicines originate from plants; however, today the awareness of the importance of being in right relationship with the plants is lost.

The earliest records of essential oil distillation go back as far as 3,000 BCE in both ancient Egypt and Pakistan. The high costs associated with the early rudimentary distillation processes of making the essential oils limited their use to aristocrats and the wealthy. The oldest medical text of ancient Egypt, the

Papyrus Ebers, dates back to 1,550 BCE and includes more than 800 essential oil medicinal formulas. In 1923 archaeologists discovered over 350 liters of preserved essential oils stored in alabaster jars inside King Tutankhamen's tomb. As advancements in technology came about, essential oils became available to the average person, emerging in the late 1900's.

The Integration of Chinese Medicine with Western Astrology and the Seasonal Cycle

Several chapters within *The Yellow Emperor's Classic of Medicine* reference the energy almanac, which corresponds to the different phases of the seasonal cycle with the acupuncture meridian system. The general overview complements the Western astrological approach to mapping the sky. Specific references associate the equinoxes and solstices with both the meridian system and meridian pathology. Classical Chinese medicine recommends treating both physical and emotional health based on the seasonal cycle used in Western astrology. Historically, Chinese medicine welcomes new concepts and technologies as long as they are supported by the fundamental governing rules. Below are the foundational pieces that support the integration of these two systems.

THE GENERAL OVERVIEW FROM CHINESE MEDICINE

"The planets within our galaxy exert the most influence on the phenomena in our world. There are further twenty-eight constellations that are observable to the naked eye in the heavens that also are significant in their import to human life. The constellations also span the entire sky, adding up to 360 degrees. With the North Star as the center of the circle in the sky, one can identify the four directions and hence each of the corresponding groups of constellations." … "Five energetic colors can be seen from the interactive movement of the constellations that correspond to the five elemental phases."

"This […the heaven is the top and the earth is the bottom… the left and the right are the space that allow for the transformation of yin and yang to take place…] has to do with the yearly cycle of the atmospheric influences. Each year there is a primary influence that affects mainly the first half of the year and that then rotates among the six influences in a given order in the years following. For convenience, imagine a wheel with the dominant influence at the top, or north, opposite the secondary influence at the bottom or south, which affects the last half of the year."[12]

"The universe potentiates change, which allows all things to manifest and prosper with unlimited energy. It also allows people to have an intelligence with which to understand the logic and reason behind all things."

When out of balance, the atmospheric influences create patterns of imbalance that affect each meridian and organ. These patterns of imbalance correspond with the Western astrological archetypes as described throughout this book.

"The change that the universe provides comes about in differing forms: in heaven there is wind on earth there is wood; in heaven there is heat, on earth there is fire; in heaven there is damp, on earth there is earth, in heaven there is dryness, on earth there is metal; in heaven there is cold, on earth there is water."

"Heaven and earth are the parameters of the existence of myriad things. Left and right are the paths of the ascending and descending yin and yang. Fire and water, heat and cold symbolize

[12] Maoshing Ni, *The Yellow Emperor's Classic of Medicine* (Boston: Shambhala, 1995), 241-242.

yin and yang. Metal [lung-Aries and large intestine-Taurus] and wood [gallbladder-Aquarius and liver-Pisces] represent the beginning and the end of life [corresponds with Western astrology and the astrological wheel]."[13]

THE SPECIFIC REFERENCES FROM CHINESE MEDICINE

The twelve branches correspond with the twelve astrological signs; however, the starting point for each system differs. The reference to the first branch starts with the first astrological sign that the Chinese New Year begins in. The Chinese New Year date fluctuates, but it always occurs during the sign of Aquarius. From this starting point, the progression of the branches matches the progression of the astrological signs. In *The Yellow Emperor's Classic of Medicine*, the description of the twelve branches from Chapter 66, The Energy Almanac, matches the seasonal cycle and the astrological archetypes as outlined below:

Third branch - first sign   *Yin* - sprouting above ground
Fourth branch - second sign   *Mao* - luxuriant vegetation in sun
Fifth branch - third sign   *Chen* - fully awakening for coming growth
Sixth branch - fourth sign   *Si* - preparation of ripeness
Seventh branch - fifth sign   *Wu* - growth as it reaches its peak
Eighth branch - sixth sign   *Wei* - sweet taste of ripeness
Ninth branch - seventh sign   *Shen* - completion and time of harvest
Tenth branch - eight sign   *You* - recollecting after rich yield
Eleventh branch - ninth sign   *Xu* - retreating from visible excitement of life
Twelve branch - tenth sign   *Hai* - seed or core awaiting next growth
First branch - eleventh sign   *Zi* - absorbing nutrients and water
Second branch - twelfth sign   *Chou* - underground growth

[13] Maoshing Ni, *The Yellow Emperor's Classic of Medicine* (Boston: Shambhala, 1995), 235-236.

Chapter 66, The Energy Almanac, also lists the time of day that each branch corresponds with. This matches the Chinese Medicine Clock and supports the corresponding progression of the astrological signs with the flow of the Chinese meridians. This same section lists the two atmospheric (heavenly) influences for each branch. When these two influences combine, they transform into one pathogenic meridian (earthly) imbalance that matches the Western astrological element associated with the corresponding sign. The energy almanac lists the associated meridian that creates the most challenging aspect for that time of year. This is the season that comes before it and strongly influences that stem's balance.

The heavenly stems correspond with the five elements and the controlling cycle in Chinese medicine. This controlling cycle follows the seasonal cycle and the natural aging process of life. The heavenly stems alternate yang (masculine) and yin (feminine) by element and each represent an aspect of the natural aging process, which follows the alternating masculine and feminine attributes of Western astrological signs.

The controlling cycle does not follow the order of the meridians by element in Chinese medicine. By associating the first stem, *Jia*, with the first sign, Aries, and adding the two luminaries (the Moon and the Sun) during their respective signs of Cancer and Leo, all twelve signs have ruling heavenly influences in an order that corresponds with the seasonal cycle and the order of the astrological signs. This provides the structure for associating the heavenly stems with the planetary rulers in Western astrology and with the associated meridians in Chinese medicine.

Aries - *Jia*: The image of breaking through, like a sprout breaking through the earth (yang-wood)

Taurus - *Yi*: The image of early growth of the young with bending stems and branches (yin-wood)

Gemini - *Bing*: The image of life force expanding like a bright beautiful fire (yang-fire)

Cancer - Transiting Moon added here

Leo - Transiting Sun added here

Virgo - *Ding*: The image of new life becoming fully grown (yin-fire)

Libra - *Wu*: The image of luxuriant growth and prosperous development (yang-earth)

Scorpio - *Ji*: The image of distinguishable features and attributes (yin-earth)

Sagittarius - *Gen*: The image of the beginning of energy reversal, energy retreating until next spring (yang-metal)

Capricorn - *Xin*: The image of withdrawing (yin-metal)

Aquarius - *Ren*: The image of life energy nurtured deeply within, like a pregnant woman nourishing a fetus (yang-water)

Pisces - *Kui*: The image of regathering a new life force, underground and invisibly cultivated, awaiting a new breakthrough (yin-water)

For example, Michelle compiled the Chinese medicine theory references for the sign of Aries: The third branch (first sign), *yin*, is the image of a crawling sprout as it meets the warmth of the air and stretches out of the earth. This corresponds with yang/wood (heat + wood = fire), the first spring month (cardinal sign), and the beginning of the day (lung meridian). The third branch (the Aries archetype) is associated with (its most challenging aspect) ministerial fire and *Shaoyang* (the triple burner or lymph system), which corresponds with the sign of Capricorn.

Astrological Sign Affirmations

ARIES
I honor who I am and my uniqueness.
I am inspired to live life to the fullest.
I take action in a careful way.

TAURUS
I am reliable and am secure in myself.
I am grounded and open to change.
I hold on to what is of value and let go of what I no longer need.

GEMINI
I am centered and focused.
I learn and grow and pace myself.
I connect and share with others in a thoughtful way.

CANCER
I honor my sensitivity and pay attention to my needs.
I nurture others and also take care of myself.
I am able to give to others from a place of fullness within.

LEO
I honor my inner fire and passion.
I live from the heart with courage.
I radiate love and joy and express my creativity.

VIRGO
I tend to the details in life in order to foster health and growth.
I see what is of value and cultivate what sustains me.
I analyze situations in order to be of service to others.

LIBRA

I am able to see my own and others' points of view.
I am committed to balance in relationships.
I am open to making changes to be fair to myself and others.

SCORPIO

I align my will with Divine will.
I dive deep into my feelings and re-surface with new insights.
I seek true empowerment for myself and others.

SAGITTARIUS

*I learn and explore in order to understand
    the deeper meaning of life.*
I am focused on my true path and purpose.
*I live with faith and hope, knowing that the sunrise
    follows the darkest night.*

CAPRICORN

I follow through on my goals in a flexible manner.
I honor my passion as well as my sense of responsibility.
I am guided by wisdom and inner knowledge.

AQUARIUS

I see the bigger picture.
I honor my commitment to truth and social justice.
I manifest my higher purpose.

PISCES

I am deeply connected with Spirit.
I trust my intuition and tune into my inner guidance.
I honor my dreams and am grounded in my reality.

Planetary / Luminary Affirmations

SUN

I am secure in who I am.
I am filled with light and life.
I live out who I am in the world.

TRANSITING SUN

I open my heart to gratitude for the present moment.
I see myself clearly and feel centered even in the midst of change.
I am open to the healing heat and light of the Sun
    to fill me with energy and uplift my spirit.

MOON

I am in tune with what I feel.
I nurture myself and am caring with others.
I am in tune with the rhythms of nature and of my body.

TRANSITING MOON

I go with the flow and stay fluid in how I deal with life.
I listen to my own rhythms and am in tune
    with the cycles of the Moon.
I honor my changing emotions and listen
    to the messages from my body.

MERCURY

I learn and think with ease.
I express myself clearly.
I move between the worlds and feel the magic of life.

VENUS A.M.

I savor the sweetness of life.
I know my worth and value myself.
I relate to others from a centered place.

VENUS P.M.

I honor my feelings and needs and those of others.
I value balance and harmony in life and in my relationships.
I reflect on my decisions and act in accordance with my values.

MARS

I act in a clear and decisive manner.
I assert myself with confidence.
I know that I am learning and growing
*   through all of my experiences.*

JUPITER

I have faith in life and feel guided and protected.
I know that life is a journey of exploration and growth.
I trust in who I am and my purpose in life.

SATURN

I grow in wisdom and am guided by Spirit.
I know who I am and my purpose, and I live that daily.
I manifest with ease.

URANUS

I strive to be an agent of positive change in the world.
I value justice and fairness.
I open my mind to the Divine mind.

NEPTUNE

I open to oneness with all of life and to Spirit.
I allow love to flow through me.
I am sensitive to others but clear with my own boundaries.

PLUTO

I align my will with Divine will.
I am open to diving deep and transforming.
I allow my life experiences to deepen my spiritual growth.

CHIRON

I am open to working on my core wounds.
I accept my vulnerabilities and am compassionate with others.
I honor my healing gifts.

Zodiac Sign Blends with Emotions

Sign	Sign Blend	Emotions in Balance	Emotions out of Balance
ARIES	40% Lemon 40% Lemon Myrtle 10% Basil 10% Peppermint	Independent Confident Inspired Foresight	Low self-esteem Mired in grief and sadness Impulsive Impatient
TAURUS	40% Jade Lemon 40% Hinoki 10% Lemon Myrtle 10% Spearmint	Grounded Practical Realistic Pragmatic Reliable	Feeling stuck Blocked Difficulties letting go Burdened
GEMINI	30% Lemon 30% Copaiba 30% Patchouli 10% Peppermint	Curious Communicative Centered	Overstimulated Spacey Scattered
CANCER	40% Tangerine 40% Fennel 10% Clove 10% Coriander	Nurturing Emotionally sensitive Secure	Overprotective Needy Worried Insecure
LEO*	40% Marjoram 40% Cypress 10% Neroli 10% Helichrysum	Joyful Courageous Loving Generous	Melancholy Depressed Self-doubting Arrogant Self-absorbed
VIRGO	30% Marjoram 30% Copaiba 20% Lavender 20% Lemon	Discerning Service-oriented Organized	Obsessed with details Self-critical Narrow-minded

*See the alternative Leo blend on page 220.

Zodiac Sign Blends with Emotions

Sign	Sign Blend	Emotions in Balance	Emotions out of Balance
LIBRA	25% Ylang ylang 25% Geranium 25% Clary sage 25% Blue spruce	Balanced Inner harmony Unselfish Caring Fair and just	Indecisive Self-sabotaging Detached Inflexible
SCORPIO	30% Ylang ylang 30% Cypress 30% Black Spruce 10% Jasmine	Strong willed Deep feelings Insightful	Self-destructive Fearful Feeling betrayed Unconscious Holds grudges Over-controlling
SAGITTARIUS	30% Cedarwood 30% Copaiba 20% Geranium 20% Cardamom	Enthusiastic Philosophical Spiritual Optimistic	Fanatical Over-zealous Lacks direction Manic
CAPRICORN	30% Cedarwood 30% Balsam Fir 30% Hinoki 10% Ledum	Living in integrity Responsible Good judgment Wise	Rigid or rule-bound Repressed emotions Tied to external expectations
AQUARIUS	30% Lavender 30% Marjoram 20% Rosemary 20% Wintergreen	Analytical Innovator Reformer Manifestor	Detached or aloof Feeling misunderstood Rebellious Fearing change
PISCES	40% Fennel 40% Orange 10% Rosemary 10% Celery seed	Mystical Spiritual High ideals Intuitive Empathic	Caught in addictions or illusions Irritable or angry Anxious Overly sensitive

Planetary / Luminary Blends with Emotions

Planet / Luminary	Planetary / Luminary Blend	Emotions in Balance	Emotions out of Balance
NATAL SUN	50% Sacred Frankincense 25% Sandalwood 25% Blue Spruce	Secure sense of self Strong vitality Sense of purpose	Poor sense of self Low energy Lacking direction or focus
TRANSITING SUN	50% Ylang Ylang 25% Sacred Frankincense 25% Frankincense	Ability to be in the present moment Clear sense of self Strong vitality	Difficulty with transitions Lack of confidence Low energy
NATAL MOON	50% Lavender 25% Black Pepper 25% Myrrh	Emotional balance Capacity to nurture self and others In tune with body and its rhythms	Moody Unaware of feelings Lack of self-care Insensitive to others Disconnected from body
TRANSITING MOON	50% Orange 25% Clove 25% Copaiba	Comfortable with change In tune with body and its rhythms Emotionally aware	Inflexible Not in touch with body Lack of emotional awareness
MERCURY	50% Grapefruit 25% Lime 25% Spearmint	Clear thinking Effective communication	Confusion Difficulty learning Communication issues

Planetary / Luminary Blends with Emotions

Planet / Luminary	Planetary / Luminary Blend	Emotions in Balance	Emotions out of Balance
VENUS AS MORNING STAR	50% Palmarosa 25% Lemongrass 25% Citronella	Enjoyment of life and beauty Strong self-worth Harmonious relationships	Lack of pleasure in life Sense of inadequacy Difficulties in relationships
VENUS AS EVENING STAR	50% Marjoram 25% Cedarwood 25% Copaiba	Discernment and strong values Strong self-worth Harmonious relationships	Lack of confidence Lack of clear values Anxiety in relationships
MARS	50% Lavender 25% Tea Tree 25% Niaouli (Melaleuca Quinquenervia)	Decisive in action Assertive	Indecisive or stuck Submissive Angry Overly aggressive
JUPITER	50% Lavender 25% Balsam Fir 25% Patchouli	Sense of faith Optimism Strong beliefs about life Self-confidence	Pessimism and hopelessness Sense that life is meaningless Overly rigid beliefs Lack of faith in self Grandiose sense of self
SATURN	50% Cypress 25% Tangerine 25% Grapefruit	Wisdom Inner strength Ability to manifest goals	Immaturity and rigidity Self-critical Controlled by external norms Blocked, unable to achieve goals

Planetary / Luminary Blends with Emotions

Planet / Luminary	Planetary / Luminary Blend	Emotions in Balance	Emotions out of Balance
URANUS	50% Marjoram 25% Rosemary 25% Tangerine	Reformer Pioneer Values diversity and equality Open to spiritual guidance	Fearful of change or rebellious Arrogant Erratic Self-absorbed
NEPTUNE	50% Bergamot 25% Geranium 25% Cardamom	Mystical, spiritual Compassionate Intuitive and empathic	Caught in addictions Mired in rescuer or victim role Emotionally overwhelmed
PLUTO	50% Cedarwood 25% Sandalwood 25% Carrot Seed	Empowered Open to transformation Deep and intense	Powerless or abusing power Lack of trust Controlling Mired in crisis and turmoil
CHIRON	50% Ylang ylang 25% Vetiver 25% Copaiba	Aware of core emotional and karmic issues Healing and compassionate with others	Mired in past wounds Self-absorbed Re-enacting painful patterns with others

Essential oils are products of nature, and their supply may be limited at times due to weather patterns, growing cycles, harvesting practices, and species scarcity. At times, you will need to use substitutions for the blends provided here. Please visit the body-feedback.com website for recommended Meramour astrology blend substitutions to go with the affirmations and acupuncture points provided in this book.

Astrology Symbols

Luminaries & Planets

☉ Sun
☽ Moon
☿ Mercury
♀ Venus
♂ Mars
♃ Jupiter
♄ Saturn
♅ Uranus
♆ Neptune
♇ Pluto
⚷ Chiron

Signs

♈ Aries
♉ Taurus
♊ Gemini
♋ Cancer
♌ Leo
♍ Virgo
♎ Libra
♏ Scorpio
♐ Sagittarius
♑ Capricorn
♒ Aquarius
♓ Pisces

Aspects

✳ Sextile
△ Trine
☌ Conjunction
☐ Square
☍ Opposition

Index

About the Authors

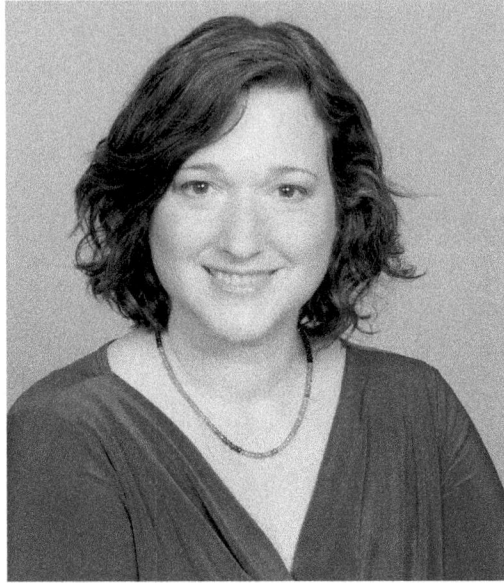

About Michelle Meramour

Michelle Meramour began her healing journey with acupuncture and holistic medicine after a severe car accident at the age of 25. While on temporary disability, Michelle started to receive acupuncture and experienced significant relief and true self-healing. After a few years, Michelle decided to change careers and help others have a better quality of life as she had experienced.

Michelle has been studying astrology since the age of 25 and often incorporates it into her treatment approach. She is an innovator in the field of acupuncture for integrating current trends in healthcare with traditional Chinese medical principles. Michelle utilizes genetic, laboratory, and muscle testing to assess health and diagnose imbalances in the acupuncture meridian system. She blends her Body-Feedback style of acupuncture with therapeutic grade essential oils, nutritional supplements, Chinese herbs, and dietary recommendations to create an individualized treatment approach.

Michelle teaches the Body-Feedback self-care techniques and educates other holistic providers in her style of acupuncture and muscle testing. She graduated Magna Cum Laude from the Midwest College of Oriental Medicine in September 2002 with a Master of Science in Oriental Medicine (MSOM). She continued her post-graduate training directly under Bob Flaws at the Blue Poppy Institute and in 2004 became certified in traditional Chinese medical gynecology.

Visit www.body-feedback.com to learn more about Michelle Meramour and her Body-Feedback techniques, or to purchase her first book, *Supporting Your Acupuncture Meridian System: How to Recover Your Health by Choosing the Best Foods, Supplements, and Essential Oils.*

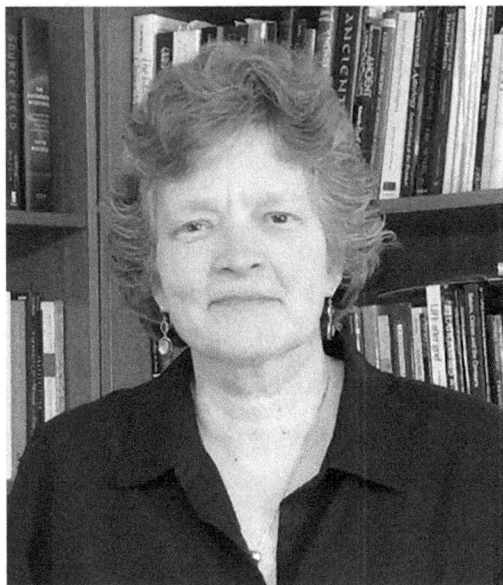

About Heather Ensworth

Heather Ensworth, Ph.D., is an internationally known astrologer who does readings with people from all over the world. She is also a clinical psychologist with over 30 years of experience. Heather has spent years studying ancient and indigenous healing traditions and is a shamanic practitioner. She has also explored many other forms of holistic healing including Chinese medicine. In addition, Heather has trained in herbalism and works with the healing energies of plants through the use of essential oils and flower essences.

Heather also has a background in cultural anthropology with a focus on ritual and symbolism and has a Masters degree in theology. She has facilitated earth-based and women's spirituality programs for over 25 years.

Heather strongly believes that to truly heal ourselves and support the healing of the Earth, we need to be in right relationship -- with ourselves, with each other, with the Earth, with the Cosmos, and with all of life.

Heather is the author of *Finding Our Center: Wisdom from the Stars and Planets in Times of Change*, IUniverse, Inc, New York, NY, 2009.

Heather can be reached through her website www.risingmoonhealingcenter.com, or by email at heather@risingmoonhealingcenter.com.

To subscribe to the Rising Moon Healing Center monthly newsletter "Currents of Change" that includes an astrological interpretation of each month's lunar cycle, contact Heather or go to the Rising Moon Healing Center website.

Heather also has a Youtube channel with information about the current astrological energies and about the profound time of transition and transformation that we are all in individually and collectively.

CPSIA information can be obtained
at www.ICGtesting.com
Printed in the USA
JSHW010138240819
1187JS00007B/20

9 780999 206904